KR_____ SAINCHUK

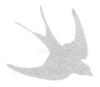

LOOSE
THREADS

Weaving Life Back Together After Cancer

Enjoy Reading!

♡ Kristy Sainchuk

"Hope. It's a powerful tool that can help us all, especially those fighting for their lives. Kristi is proof that hope works, and she reminds us all that we are not alone, even when we think all hope is lost. Her strength is inspiring."

– Rob Williams, Cohost, CTV Morning Live Edmonton

"Whether the diagnosis is yours or of someone you love, *Loose Threads* is a transformational read for everyone in your circle. Kristi's anecdotes, advice, and straightforward style are simultaneously soothing and empowering."

– Shannon Tyler, Radio and Television Personality

"Knowing someone with cancer is very different from knowing how they live with it, or more importantly, how they survive it. Kristi Sainchuk describes her journey with intense and raw honesty and shares how the battle with cancer impacts an entire family. *Loose Threads* is a book not just about surviving cancer, but thriving in spite of it. Powerful.

– Jason Gregor, President, Just a Game Production and host of The Jason Gregor Show on TSN 1260

"As someone who has experienced cancer first hand, Kristi uses her diagnosis as a platform for frank, honest conversation. Her book recounts her experiences and enlightens those who face similar challenges using practical solutions."

– Elissa Woolnough, educator, breast cancer survivor

"After years of being an advocate for women struggling through cancer treatment and its aftermath, I know *Loose Threads* is a must read for anyone and everyone who has faced this devastating disease. This book is a roadmap for both those with a diagnosis and loved ones supporting their beloved warriors. May we all be as heroic and share such details of our epic struggle in hopes of making it easier for those who have been there and have yet to follow."

– Donna Yost, Best-dressed Author and Inspiration

Editorial Project Management: Karen Rowe, www.karenrowe.com

Cover Design: Kurt Richmond, kurt.richmond@oddballdesignz.com

Inside Layout: Ljiljana Pavkov

Printed in the United States

ISBN: 978-1-9991776-0-7 (paperback)

ISBN: 978-1-9991776-1-4 (ebook)

For My Dad,

Thank you for teaching me that time
is never up.

"In the midst of winter, I found there was, within me, an invincible summer [...] For it says that no matter how hard the world pushes against me, within me, there's something stronger – something better, pushing right back."

– Albert Camus

Table of Contents

Foreword by Todd Herman 13

Note to the Reader 17

Introduction 19

Chapter 1: The Diagnosis 25

Chapter 2: Chemotherapy 35

Chapter 3: The Side Effects 51

Chapter 4: Chemo, Kids, and Loneliness 65

Chapter 5: Support Systems 73

Chapter 6: Mastectomy, Menopause, and More 85

Chapter 7: Radiation 99

Chapter 8: Bloody and Bandaged, but Beautiful .. 105

Chapter 9: Professional and Social Support 111

Chapter 10: Weave It Out 133

Chapter 11: What's Different in My Life Because
    of Cancer 147

Chapter 12: Who I am Now 159

Acknowledgements 165

About the Author 169

LOOSE
THREADS

Weaving Life Back Together After Cancer

Foreword

by Todd Herman

We all go on a hero's journey and sometimes you can choose to be the hero and other times you are an accidental hero.

Kristi Sainchuk was an accidental hero. From diagnosis, chemotherapy, radiation, treatment, a double mastectomy, and beyond, Kristi was willing to accept her situation and thrive as a result of it. Even though Kristi didn't choose to have cancer, she chose not to see herself as a victim. And when you do that, you free your mental space up to start thinking in a healthier way. You can find solutions, support and a better attitude.

When adversity hits you, what are you going to do with it?

1997 was the first time I met Kristi. I was standing in the kitchen at a restaurant in Edmonton, Alberta, Canada. She was a server and I was a chef's apprentice. This sassy little punk came into the back and was throwing some shade and trash talk our way.

Of course, I liked her immediately.

Every time I had a chance to talk to Kristi, it felt like a quasi-standup comedy routine. Her humour and sarcasm are what endeared me towards her. And what has caused us to be close friends for 25 years.

Shortly after we met I started a peak performance training company. For 22 years, we've focused on helping professional athletes, Olympic athletes, CEOs, leaders and entrepreneurs develop the focus, mindset, and discipline to win in their pursuits. We've conducted research and clocked over 30,000 hours working with people creating extraordinary results. I have spoken on hundreds of stages around the world and wrote the Wall Street Journal bestselling book: *The Alter Ego Effect: The Power of Secret Identities to Transform Your Life*.

The only reason I mention it, is because I've seen good people, with tough situations, do incredible things. And the book your holding will allow you to see yourself in Kristi's journey, so you can do the same.

The things that drive people are often complex and nuanced. Life will always bump you up against obstacles. Whether they are chosen or get thrust upon you by no choice of your own. If you're reading this book, chances are you've been put into a volatile and uncertain situation you didn't choose. Often, an identity crisis can take place and many people fall into a depressive state or end up dealing with issues around mental health.

This is doubly so with a cancer diagnosis.

Remember, Cancer is not your entire identity.

My hope throughout the course of this book is you begin to see your situation as an opportunity for a reinvention and a rebirth. Resisting the situation will prevent you from seeing what is on the other side: a newer, stronger, better version of yourself.

As I read the story on the following pages, I was struck with the power of the human spirit. We all enter the fire. But what do we do with that fire? Do we get burned or do we forge new steel in that fire? Kristi's story is all about new steel being forged.

Over the years I have helped tens of thousands of people achieve their most ambitious goals by becoming more creative, confident and courageous. These are all traits I saw in Kristi early on that I know served her well throughout her cancer journey. I am so inspired to see her pass along these tools to other women and families dealing with a breast cancer diagnosis.

As you walk through your own fire, I encourage you to focus on your greatest power within, your ability to choose who shows up. Because on the other side of this transformation is someone you'll be proud to meet. Just like I'm proud to know Kristi and get the chance to write a few words in this powerful story you hold.

Todd Herman,
Author of the bestselling book, *The Alter Ego Effect: The Power of Secret Identities to Transform Your Life.*, Performance Coach, & Entrepreneur.
New York, New York

Note to the Reader

This book is intended as a quick reference guide for those affected by a cancer diagnosis. It can either be read from start to finish, or you can jump straight to the relevant section. As such, those that choose to read from start to finish may notice some repetition. This was intentionally left to support our readers who may be short on time, attention, energy, patience, or all of the above.

This is the book I wish had been written when I was first diagnosed, and I hope it will help you as much as writing it has helped me.

Take what works for you and leave the rest.

Introduction

I was thirty-six years old when I started as the personal stylist for Southgate Center, a shopping mall in Edmonton, Alberta, Canada. In this high-fashion job, I was helping women look and feel their best, attending store openings and getting invited to lavish events. It was my dream job.

At home, I was mother to amazing two-year-old twins, to whom I had given birth through in vitro fertilization (IVF). I was happily married to an incredible husband, who was running nightclubs and driven to succeed and provide for his family. He was a man in the know, and we were living the life!

But that was all on the outside. Inside, a war was being raged against my body, though I didn't know it at the time. There were signs that my life wasn't as perfect as it seemed, but I never made the connection. At twenty-four years old, I suddenly started getting debilitating migraines, which continued for years. My kids were angel babies, but as anyone with toddlers—and especially twins—can attest, they could cause high stress. When you have twins, you have double the hormones going through your body so my emotions were out of whack.

But that wasn't the only reason for my emotional and mental tumult. When the twins were only ten months old, I got pregnant again. I was thrilled to be having another child, but naturally, my husband Mike and I were also concerned by the additional strain a third child would bring to our already complicated lives. As it turned out, we never had the opportunity to adapt to a growing family. The pregnancy was ectopic, meaning the fetus was developing in one of my fallopian tubes, rather than in the uterus. I found out about ten weeks into my pregnancy, when I experienced the most excruciating pain of my life.

My tube burst, spawning an intense amount of internal bleeding. Not only did I lose my child, but I almost died. The experience was traumatic, to say the least. And in retrospect, I realized I never properly grieved that loss—not on my own, nor with my husband.

My reasons to grieve only compiled when, ten months later, I lost my best friend Jen to a car accident. She was in a car that hit a patch of black ice. Cruelly, this was the same way my grandparents had died when I was sixteen years old, and this additional loss triggered that age-old trauma I hadn't known how to properly process the first time around.

On the inside, my emotions spun deeper and deeper into a dangerous cycle of negative rumination and despair. On the outside, I felt like I was supposed to be okay with everything that had happened. I kept an appearance of control. I felt in control of my work. As a parent, I felt in control of my two kids. I was hyper-focused on details I could control. But when something didn't go according to my plan, I didn't know how to handle it and would often spiral out of control.

I knew I was experiencing depression. I had already gone to the doctor prior to Jen's death and had been put on medication for post-partum depression. But I didn't understand that I'd been through a series of traumas that I needed to address and heal. I also needed to start implementing a regular and regimented self-care routine.

But I continued with daily life as if nothing had happened. I would get up early in the morning, get the kids ready, and drop them off at daycare. Then, I'd go to work, pick them up at the end of the day, and bring them along to meet whomever I had promised to meet for coffee that day. Every column in my day-calendar was filled either with driving, working, or socializing until I went to bed. This is how I thought it was supposed to be.

I was so busy filling my time with people-pleasing and constantly worrying about being late that my own needs got pushed to the back burner. I would never dream of cancelling, and I rarely, if ever, put my own needs first. I remember one day thinking I felt spread thin like butter and needed to slow my life down.

I wouldn't even let people come to me; I would always do everything I could for them, even though I was the one who probably needed the love and support. I wasn't self-aware enough at that time to realize and therefore didn't know how to slow down or ask for help. My life had become a knot of tightly woven fabric with no room for the light to shine in.

At the beginning of 2012, my husband and I took the kids and the nanny on a vacation to Maui. There I was in one of the most beautiful places on earth, and I could not get out of bed. All I wanted to do was sleep all day. That was when I realized something was deeply wrong. I returned home and thought, *I can't go on living like this. I think my kids might be better off without me. I'm a disaster.* I remember one night, in particular, just sitting in the darkness of my house while everyone was asleep thinking, *I just want everything to stop.*

Life as I knew it did entirely come to a stop when, about two months after returning from Hawaii, I discovered a lump on my breast. At thirty-six years old, cancer was not part of my plan. My plan was to be a fashionista with two fashionable kids. That plan – along with everything else in my life I thought I had under control – began to unravel.

Cancer would be the end of my world as I knew it, but it was certainly not the end of the world. It was the start of learning how to weave my life back together, this time allowing space for the light to get through. In 2012 I was undergoing chemotherapy. Now, among many other beautiful things, I teach children and adults about Saori weaving; I talk to those that ask about mental health. And, of course, I wrote this book so that you too can see that a cancer diagnosis doesn't mean you are going to die. It may just mean you will be rewoven.

Chapter 1:

The Diagnosis

It was a Tuesday. Like any mother of two-and-a-half-year-old twins, I was working through the mountain of toddler laundry in my house. While walking across my kitchen with a laundry basket under my arm, something in the way I moved prompted me to put my hand on my chest. I thought to myself, *Huh, that's not supposed to be there*. I felt a lump.

My doctor had always told me, "Think of your breast as spaghetti and sauce; you're always going to feel stuff in there moving around. But if you ever feel a meatball, that's when you need to come see me." This was a meatball.

Never in my wildest dreams did I ever think I would have breast cancer at thirty-six years old. There was no breast cancer in my family, but I knew I needed to get the lump checked out. Luckily, I already had a doctor's appointment scheduled for the following day to get some prescriptions refilled. I went to my appointment, and at the end of the visit I said, "Oh, and there's this thing you should maybe check out."

I had known my doctor since I was eighteen years old. She has treated my whole family. Because I have such a strong relationship with her and she knows my personality, when I came to her with the lump she said, "This might be nothing, but it might be something. And if it's something, I want you to know that your head's going to spin because it will all go so fast." She was already preparing me, but in a nice way, for news that I had cancer. She made a recommendation for a mammogram, and I made an appointment for the following week.

That whole week, I kept thinking, *It's probably nothing, just a swollen gland or whatever*. But at the same time, my mind was swirling with the thought, *It could be breast cancer*. Ironically, what I was most concerned about was my job. I had a huge presentation to give in a week and a half. I thought, *If I have all these tests to do, I won't be able to do my job!* The only person I confided in was Jenny, who had hired me at Southgate Centre and happened to be my friend. I was the Head Fashion Stylist there; I knew I could trust her to keep things to herself. I didn't want to worry anybody over nothing (because this was probably nothing).

Leading up to the day of the mammogram, my parents decided to come into town and stay overnight with us. I didn't want to worry them with news of a lump, but I had never asked my mom about the history of cancer on her side of the family. I decided to tell her I was having a mammogram and that I had found a lump (that was probably nothing). She told me there was not a lot of cancer on her side of the family, except for my maternal grandfather having lip cancer. This was good news to me. I couldn't have breast cancer. I'm young with no family history of it, and did I mention I'm young?

I asked my husband to come with me on the day of my mammogram, "the big M." They gave me a breast-cancer-pink robe to wear and told me to squeeze my breast into a machine. They squeezed that machine until it hurt. Next was an ultrasound, and then I was sent to the waiting room while the radiologist looked at the results of the tests.

They're just going to come back and tell me it was nothing, I thought. But instead, the nurse came back and said, "Can you come in first thing in the morning? We need to do a biopsy." At that point, I figured the news wasn't good but still hoped that they simply needed to eliminate cancer as a possibility. So, the next morning I went in and was given four biopsies— one in my right breast (the one without the lump) and three in my left. As they worked their way around the lump, it felt like they were using a staple gun with four or five needles. It's a very rude procedure.

Meanwhile, nobody was talking to me. I had no idea what was going on. They were testing so many different spots in the breast, and I only had one lump. I was really confused. Finally, I asked the technician what was going on. She said to me, "We are checking into the calcifications you have around your nipple, the lump you have, and a few lymph nodes on the left side. On the right, you may have a blocked milk duct. We just want to make sure that you never have to come back here." She was holding my hand at the time. The way everyone was acting was giving me an indication that something bad was happening.

They told me I'd have to wait five days before getting my results back, and I would get a call from my doctor. That reaffirmed my fear. I'd had ultrasounds before. If nothing was wrong, they would say, "Everything's fine." I'd get a wink and a nudge as I'd go out the door. This time I didn't get that. I started crying before I left the room. The technician got my husband to console me. I was terrified it was something, but a small part of me still believed it could be nothing.

Having to wait those five days for the test results was extremely hard. Nobody had said I had breast cancer yet, but I started to think that I did. I tried to keep myself busy with the kids and my work and still tried to tell myself it was nothing right up until I got the call from my doctor. She wanted me to come into her office for the results. By then, I pretty much knew what she was going to tell me.

I was with my husband when my doctor came in. She threw open the door and said, "There's no easy way to say this. You have breast cancer." She just ripped it off like a Band-Aid, which I think is one of the best things she's ever done for me. It would have been worse if she had dragged the news out. I didn't want handholding or pity. Giving it to me gently wouldn't have changed the result.

I started to cry, and my husband started to cry. It was all a blur. She gave me directions. I had to go see this other doctor at the cancer care centre for my region, known as the Cross Cancer Institute. She walked me through what was going to happen next, but all I could think was, *Oh my god, I'm going to die.*

As I was leaving, I asked, "Does this mean I'm going to die?"

She held my shoulders, looked me straight in the eyes and said, "No, this doesn't mean you're going to die." I trusted her when she said that. I took her words to heart and knew I was going to be okay. But I also knew it wasn't going to be easy.

Dealing with the Diagnosis – It's not my job to cure cancer

One of the worst things about getting a cancer diagnosis for a people-pleaser like me is having to tell the people you love. I didn't want to make them sad. I was more worried about my family and my job than I was about having cancer. I phoned my mom and dad on the way home from the hospital. After I got home, I called Jenny from work. I told her I had gotten my results back, and I had breast cancer. I was still worried about my work, and I told her I didn't think I could do my big presentation the next day. In hindsight, it's incredible to me that I still had a concern about not letting anyone down. She was so understanding and of course, told me not to worry about work. Jenny has since told me that she hung up the phone with me that day and burst into tears.

I was in shock. I didn't have time for Cancer.

After making the necessary phone calls and telling some of my friends about my diagnosis, I was left with my thoughts. Naturally, they were all about cancer. Cancer had always been, to me, the worst thing that could ever happen to anybody. It was my worst fear ever that I would get it, and now I had it.

An analysis that I came up with for my sanity was that typically when someone gets sick, they go to the doctor and get a prescription. Usually in less than a week, whatever they have goes away. Cancer is an awful, horrible, terrible, monster of a disease so the prescription for cancer is a horrible, monstrous solution.

Instead of taking seven pills and being done in a week, I would have to go through all these horrible, terrible things like chemotherapy, radiation, and losing a body part. Treatment may last for a year or longer, but there is treatment. Coming to terms with that reality is what helped me. The alternative would be thinking, *Oh my God, there's no cure for cancer, and I'm going to die*. That was just too existential to think about. I didn't have time to think about leaving my twins without a mom. Those two little people needed me. I never thought of it as positive thinking; I thought of it as a necessary aspect of parenting – reframing the thought of cancer to make it more doable so I could be around to watch my kids grow up.

The other tool that helped me was knowing that cancer was completely out of my control. Once I realized that it was so beyond my control, I stopped worrying about it because *it wasn't my job to cure cancer.* That was someone else's job. My job was to get better. If I thought that I could cure it, then I would have wasted time on the Internet every day obsessing over information than ultimately would have made my situation worse. My energy and focus would have been scattered, chasing down potential hair-brained or unsuccessful solutions. Instead, I chose to listen to doctors who had proven, effective treatments. Oncologists, the doctors that treat cancer, in particular go to school for many years to learn about cancer and how to treat it. They must complete up to 13 years of training, including an undergraduate degree, a medical degree, a residency, and an optional fellowship. This was their job.

Making those mental shifts gave me time to worry about little things that I *did* have control over—like what I was going to eat for lunch, what my kids were doing, how my kids were doing, what I was going to wear to chemo (Hey, I'm a fashion stylist!), or who was going to bring me chocolate and ice cream when I was feeling down. Slowly, my tightly-woven mind began to soften—because it had to. All of the perfectly-aligned threads that had made up my life—the plans that filled up my hourly, daily, and monthly calendar—had to be allowed to stretch and breathe and alter course.

Interestingly, finding out that I had cancer snapped me out of my depression. The medication I was on kept my feelings about my mortality at a distance. That was a blessing in a way. With cancer in the periphery of my brain rather than written all over my face, I could handle my day-to-day life.

When thoughts about my mortality did come up, I asked myself what that would look like. I pictured myself in the hospital, with my husband and the kids at my bedside. I asked myself how I felt. Was I scared? No. Was I sad? Nope. I kept worrying that I was in denial about being sick because I wasn't terrified every day about dying. I don't know if it's because of the drugs I was on, making my emotions less palpable, but I was only sad for my family. When I died, I wouldn't have to worry about cancer anymore. I was sad for my kids and my husband, but for me it would be over. My husband and I never talked about what would happen if I died. We didn't discuss living wills or power of attorney. We always put that conversation on the back burner, thinking if we talked about it, then it would happen.

I just resolved that I had a shitty disease, I'd have to take some horrible medicine for a long time, but I was going to get through it. The first part of my "prescription" was chemotherapy—eight rounds over six months. The second part was a radical mastectomy. The third part was radiation. If I did those things, then I would be okay. It might not take five days, like with the flu, but maybe in a year, the cancer would be gone. That narrative really helped me, and maybe it will help you or someone you love too.

Chapter 2:

Chemotherapy

When I met with my oncologist for the first time, I brought my husband and my sister-in-law, who was a nurse, with me to record notes. I was given a phone number when I went to the Cross Cancer Institute that I could call to speak with a nurse with any questions I had after the visit. The nurse could also review the information from the visit with me—what type of cancer I had, what my treatment plan would be, the two types of chemotherapy I would have, and so on. There was no way I would have been able to retain everything I was told, or even understand it, while under emotional duress.

When people hear "breast cancer," they usually have a general idea in mind as to what that means—cancer that has originated in the tissue of the breast, in layman's terms. But there are many different kinds of breast cancer. The most common type is genetic breast cancer; it's called BRCA1 or BRCA2, and it occurs when someone inherits it from their mother, aunt, or another relative.

The second type that is most commonly heard about is HER2-positive cancer, which is hormone receptor-positive cancer. With this type, there are receptors on the outside of a cancer cell, and when certain hormones touch that cell, it turns on and starts to replicate itself over and over again. However, there is a treatment for this type of cancer—a drug called Herceptin, which I'll talk more about later.

The type that I was first diagnosed with was estrogen receptor-positive cancer. This cancer has receptor cells on the outside as well, but when estrogen touches that cell, it decides that it is a good time to divide and conquer and become "big cancer." My prescription for this type of cancer is a drug I've been placed on for ten years called Tamoxifen. This drug shuts off all the estrogen production in my body. Cancer cells can linger in the body—even after chemotherapy and radiation—but dormant cells usually don't live past ten years. It's a very harsh drug to be on for so long, and a lot of people can't tolerate it. I'm one of the lucky few that can.

At the time I was diagnosed, there was no real history of cancer or breast cancer in my family. My paternal uncle died from pancreatic cancer; he was the only one to have the disease. Cancer wasn't a big word in my household. It wasn't something I knew anything about, and that was a really scary place to be because all I associated it with was Terry Fox—the Canadian athlete and cancer activist who died from the disease. Therefore, my thoughts went immediately to, *I'm going to die.*

My cancer was not genetic. I had all the testing for it done not just for my own sake, but because I was worried about my daughter. I don't have the genes, but still, my doctors recommended that my daughter get tested for it ten years before the age I was diagnosed at; she'll have to start going for mammograms at twenty-six, just to make sure.

Two years after I got cancer, my mother-in-law got breast cancer. Two years after that, my maternal aunt got breast cancer, and two years after that, my mom got breast cancer. But I still didn't have genetic breast cancer.

The Early Days

I assumed the first step in my treatment for breast cancer would be surgery, but that was a common misconception. First, I had to have several more tests—a bone scan, a chest x-ray, and an MRI (or CT scan). The goal was to determine if the cancer had metastasized and turned into stage four cancer.

After waiting another five days for the results from those three tests, I received a call from my general surgeon at 6 a.m. one morning. "I'm happy to tell you that you're stage three. I thought you would want to know that as early as possible," she shared. After that good news, I was told that chemotherapy was the first step in my treatment plan. The goal with the first round was to test if it would work by attempting to shrink my tumor; the result would determine the rest of my treatment.

At the time of diagnosis, I didn't know anyone who had cancer, let alone breast cancer. But I knew my friend's dad had had cancer, and he'd also done some volunteering at the Cross Cancer Institute. This friend was one of the first people I'd phoned and she said, "You should call my dad." So, I did, and it was probably one of the best decisions I made at that point. He made a lot of my fears go away.

He told me there were three different rooms that I would have chemotherapy in; two on the main floor, and one on the fourth floor. He said, "It doesn't matter what cancer you have or what treatment you have, they just put you wherever there's room. So, don't jump to conclusions—it doesn't mean you're worse off if you're on the fourth floor or better off if you're on the first floor or in the dayroom."

That was really valuable information. He also told me that the nurses that work in the chemotherapy ward would be there for me and that no question is stupid. "They want to know how you're feeling the minute you get one drip of chemotherapy in your veins," he said. "They want to know if the hair on your head stands up or you get an irregular heartbeat, or your skin feels weird. This helps them determine if you're going to have an allergic reaction to the drug. Tell them everything that's going on with you. You are never bugging them."

Something else important that he shared was, "People aren't going to know how to help you. You're going to have somebody show up at your house with food that maybe you don't feel like eating, because you're going to be nauseous. All you have to do is say thank you. And if you go and throw that soup away, that's fine; they don't need to know. But that is all people can do for you."

He also told me that, because most chemotherapies are in three-week cycles, my body would go through a somewhat predictable cycle. For example, on day one of getting chemotherapy, I might not feel so bad, but on day five or six, I would feel really bad—perhaps really nauseated. Then at around day ten or eleven, my immune system would go down; that's when all I would want to do was stay in bed. Then by day fifteen, I'd feel better and my taste would start to come back. (The minute I'd start with chemotherapy, I'd get a metallic taste in my mouth that made everything I ate taste awful. My friend's dad tipped me off—"Don't eat things you really like, because it's going to ruin them for you.") Again, really valuable advice. I'm happy to report that I still love pizza.

With this kind of insight from someone who had been through what I was going through, I was able to feel better. I thought, *He got through it, so I can get through it.* It made me wonder, *Why don't they put this in a pamphlet somewhere?!*

They did give me pamphlets, but of course, they weren't all-inclusive. I even had to take a class in advance about chemotherapy. The instructor explained that the drugs we were going to take would kill the fastest-growing cells in our bodies, which are cancer cells. But they also kill the cells on the inside of our mouths, the cells in our intestines, our whole digestive tract from top to tail, and our hair cells. That's why we would lose our hair.

In the class, we were given reading material that suggested a high-calorie, high-protein diet. My brothers used to tease me and say that if I were having grilled cheese, put extra cheese on it. If I was having jam on my toast, put extra jam. As a joke, they bought me mini packets of maple syrup to put on everything I ate while I was in chemo so I could get those extra calories.

My Chemo Experience

I knew in advance that I would have to take a lot of heavy drugs. I was a little bit fearful of that because my brother was going through nursing school at the time. When I gave him the names of the drugs I would be on, he said, "Those are all on the restricted drug list. They're going to put those in your body?!" Yup. I began to assume I'd go into chemo, and the nurse would be in a full hazmat suit putting me through the wringer.

They prepared my body for the attack a couple of days in advance of chemotherapy with three or four anti-nausea drugs taken at various intervals. I had a friend who was a pharmacist, and once I got all my chemotherapy drugs, all the anti-nausea drugs, and my treatment plan, I sent him the list. He warned me, "Once you get nauseous and start throwing up, it's really hard to get back to normal. They're going to give you the anti-nausea drugs to take the day before, the day of, and the day after. And then they give you another set of drugs to take as needed. Take those **before** you get nauseated, before you need them." I took that advice to heart and always started the "to be taken as needed drugs" as soon as my other anti-nausea drugs were done.

Therefore, once all of my main drugs ran out during the first three days of chemo, I took the anti-nausea medicine every four hours for ten days. I think I only threw up once throughout all of my treatments! I learned that I could also talk to my pharmacist, who could sometimes share more information about the drugs than my oncologists.

Since I had been on antidepressants and medication for migraines for years before that, I wasn't afraid of taking drugs. But I wasn't thrilled at the idea of taking Intravenous (IV) drugs. For my treatment, I was to have eight rounds of chemotherapy, four rounds of one cocktail and then four rounds of another cocktail, and I'd have three weeks in between each of those chemotherapies. They were 21-day treatments. I started April 3rd and would be done on September 11th, 2012.

To prepare for my first day of chemo, I packed a book bag with several books, cards, and games. I expected I'd be there for several hours. My husband

came with me. When I first arrived, the nurse intro-
duced herself, and I handed her my check-in sheet.
It included all the information about myself, my diagnosis, medications, and treatment. Every time I went
into chemo, I would get asked several times, "Is this
your name? What's your birthday? What's your E number?" Every cancer patient at the Institute gets an "E"
number. It's a number that is unique to every individual. When staff members come to administer chemotherapy, they want to make sure they are giving each
patient the correct treatment.

Then I was asked, "Do you need a warm blanket?"
I told her I did. She asked if I also wanted a hot pack.

I asked, "What's a hot pack?" She handed me
one; it's basically a sealed hot water bottle. They had
me place it on my arm to prepare my veins for the
IV. Although it serves a functional purpose, it also felt
cozy and warm. *This isn't so bad*, I thought.

She continued casually, "Okay, I'm going to be right
back. We're going to make sure your drugs are here,
so sit tight." The staff members were so lovely and
knowledgeable. It eased some of my anxiety, knowing
it was just business as usual for them.

The nurse came back to get me and said, "Okay,
we're going to put you in this bed over here, follow
me." When I first walked into the chemotherapy
room, I had the worst feeling. There were so many
people hooked up to machines with bags of medicine. Some people were by themselves, and others had loved ones with them. It hit me how serious

my situation was; I felt it was going to be really dire. *This is cancer*, I thought. *I've got to put my serious glasses on because this is it.*

But then she brought me into a side room, and it was brightly colored with a mural of a hot air balloon. There were three beds, and I was the first person in the room. Before long two more breast cancer patients joined me. I thought, *Okay, everyone's going to stay to themselves. No one's going to be talking.*

But instead, one of the ladies who was getting her IV started staring at my husband and said, "Let's see your tattoos. We want to see your tattoos." He obliged and started the show. We just became a group of women, bonding and having a good time instead of approaching the experience with the mindset, *We're having chemo. This is serious business.*

The drug I was to receive was called Epirubicin. It was the color of cherry Kool-Aid. The nurse brought over eight vials, big giant syringes, and said, "Okay, I have to push this in. We can't let it go through the drip."

Being curious, I asked, "Why not?"

And she explained, "Because if there's some sort of leak and it goes anywhere outside of your vein, it will cause necrosis of the tissue." In other words, whatever it touched would die. That's what they were putting in me to kill cancer. For forty-five minutes, she slowly pushed the drug into my veins, watching it carefully. By the end of all of my chemotherapy treatments, that drug would turn my veins into violin strings. It hurt to straighten my arm or carry anything.

Another nurse told me, "If you're having this kind of chemo, you should have some ice with you because when you take this drug, having ice in your mouth decreases the side effects." They knew everything! And they did indeed want to know anything and everything that happened to me throughout the process. If they put in my IV and it hurt just a smidge, they wanted to know. "Okay, we'll fix that. No problem," they'd say.

The saving grace of going through chemotherapy at the Cross is that they have amazing volunteers. Every time I went there for chemo, there would be this little cart that came by every couple of hours, pushed by two volunteers. They had tea, coffee, orange juice, apple juice, and free cookies for everybody having chemo. As small as a free cookie and tea seem, they were honestly the best things I had to look forward to while getting chemo. I was always wondering, *Where's the volunteer cart? I need my free cookie.*

I thought I'd want to read to pass some time, but I always got really sleepy and really cold. I'd always accept the offer of the warm blanket, straight out of the toaster oven, or whatever they used to keep them warm! With that, I slept through most of my chemo sessions, although I'd always have somebody there with me. It wasn't always my husband; my mom came with me once, and various friends helped out.

All the staff at the Cancer Institute in the chemotherapy department are wonderful human beings.

They never made me feel like I was getting the worst chemicals ever in my body. They would say, "You're just going to get a little medicine here." That put me at ease.

The chemotherapy worked. It didn't get rid of the tumor completely, but it managed to shrink it considerably from two centimeters down to 0.8 centimeters. The next step would be surgery.

I want to mention that in Canada, we are lucky to have public healthcare. I recognize that a major concern for American or uninsured cancer patients is the cost treatment entails. I can't speak for all of the different insurance systems and costs involved, but I can say that there was one drug that went beyond my healthcare coverage that was ridiculously expensive.

On day one of my twenty-one day cycle of chemo, I would go to the Cross and they would do bloodwork. If my platelets, red blood cells, and white blood cells were all at a certain level—making me healthy enough to have chemo—I would get chemo the next day. If I didn't have strong enough white blood cells, I would have to wait a week or two until I was strong enough to get chemo again. The problem is, that gives cancer another week or two to grow, which nobody wants. Instead of waiting, I was given the option of injecting a shot of Neulasta at home. Then, I would wait a week and if I was healthy enough, I'd have chemo, or else I'd have to take the drug again. Throughout treatment, I had to inject this drug six times—at $2,000 a shot.

My healthcare covered 70% of my drug coverage, but only to a $10,000 a year limit. I basically ate up my entire drug coverage for the year with one drug and was still charged $2,000. Thankfully, the Cross has a "bridge program" that helped pay for this uncovered portion. The sad part is, if someone can't afford that drug, then their chemo treatment has to be watered down, making it less effective.

I would oftentimes look around at the Cross and see people in less fortunate circumstances than my own. I was grateful that I could afford to have cancer, financially and emotionally. I had the funds to pay for a wig, Neulasta, and my everyday bills. And I had a ton of support from friends and family. I had a husband with the flexibility in his schedule to accompany me to chemo, the drive to work so hard to support us, and the energy to double down on parenting when I was really sick. But that is not always the case for everyone. I would see people getting chemo and going to appointments by themselves. Being sick is a very lonely place to be, at the best of times.

What I Wish I Had Known

When I lost my hair, I didn't just lose my hair. My head started to hurt because my hair follicles were dying. I had never heard that this was a sign that my hair was starting to fall out. Also, it doesn't all fall out at once;

mine fell out in a way that made me look like a clown. I had a weird male-pattern balding going on. I would lose my hair fully on the crown of my head but on the sides and back, it would be patchy and thin. Nothing screams attractive like feeling you need to have a combover. What a fashionista! That's why I shaved it (down to the wood, as they say), and I would get it shaved every couple of weeks. Not only was it one of the few things I could control, but it made it look like I had a cute little bald head. I needed all the help I could get to feel somewhat normal.

I got mouth sores. No one told me about that. All I heard about was nausea and throwing up. As an adult migraine sufferer for 10 years, the nausea from chemo didn't feel that much different from a migraine, and I didn't have nausea from chemo that often. What I did have was a mouth that was on fire, so much that I could hardly eat. My teeth hurt. My gums hurt. Everything in my mouth hurt. I had to use a special prescription mouthwash.

Because of the pain in my mouth, I didn't have much of an appetite, so I ate a lot of macaroni and cheese, chicken noodle soup, or toast—things that were bland. But even toast was almost too sharp for my mouth, so I ate buns with butter. I drank a lot of ginger ale. I remember a time when a friend came over and made me one of my favorite meals, a beautiful salad with beets, goat cheese, rotisserie chicken, and almonds. I just couldn't eat it because my mouth was too sore. #realitiesofchemo

My hands and feet were on fire all the time. The drug, Docetaxel made my fingers and toes hurt. I lost my fingernails and my toenails. And my fingernails didn't even look like fingernails; they were splitting down the middle. By the end of chemo, I had lost the feeling in the tips of my fingers and toes. I had a hard time walking in heels and knowing where my feet were going to land. Yes, I wore wedge sandals. It was the end of summer, and I wanted to feel beautiful. To say the least, my hands and feet looked like they had been through the wringer.

I also didn't know that I wouldn't be able to go outside and spend a lot of time with others. I wasn't supposed to be around children because my immune system was so low. I didn't cut myself off from people though, because being around others gave me some sense of normalcy. I made sure on the days that my immune system was the lowest to stay to myself and only be around healthy individuals. I did not want to be sicker than I already was.

One thing people don't necessarily think about in advance is that if you don't have a car or you're not fit to drive back home, how do you get to and from chemo? Thankfully, I had a lot of people offer to take me, but there are also volunteers that will do that. Just as there were volunteers scheduled to bring tea and cookies to chemo patients, there were volunteers at the Cross who were available to drive patients to appointments or bring an "art cart" to supply materials for knitting or coloring while waiting for appointments (anything to take their minds off cancer!)

Something else I wish I had known is that, if you are a new cancer patient, what's important to note is that, even if you have the same kind of cancer as somebody else, it doesn't mean you're going to get the same treatment as someone else. Your treatments are specific to you. Some of the chemo treatments are the same for different types of cancers, but most everything is tailored to you. You are going to react to the drugs differently than someone else. I didn't have a lot of allergic reactions to my treatments, but a lot of people do.

If you have cancer, my suggestion is to listen to your body as you're getting chemotherapy. If you have questions about what you're experiencing, ask a nurse. There are no dumb questions. There's a hotline you can always call and talk to a nurse who will answer everything that you ask. Use what is available to you, because otherwise, it can feel like you are venturing into the unknown.

What I thought was going to happen is that I would end up in a recliner, feeling like Walter White on *Breaking Bad*. But chemotherapy ended up being a somewhat social experience. I had one lady tell me her whole cancer story as I sat there. I listened to her as she said, "You're lucky you caught yours early. I didn't catch mine so early. I was scared to go." That's when I realized people are really scared to go to the doctor.

She thought something was wrong but waited years to get it diagnosed. Early detection is really important!

Finally, don't compare your experience with anyone else's and don't make assumptions. For example, your friend's treatment may take a long time, but yours might not. Experiences are very different based on several factors, including the type of cancer one has. I have a friend with cervical cancer whose chemo treatment took eight hours; whereas, mine took about three hours. I also have a friend who had non-Hodgkin's lymphoma. He'd go in for a treatment for two days, but then he wouldn't come back until months later for a type of "maintenance" chemo. Everyone's different.

My mom won the lottery of cancers. She didn't have to have chemotherapy. Instead, she had a lumpectomy, a surgery where only a portion of the breast is removed, and radiation. I was so happy for her because for me chemotherapy was the hardest part. For others, however, radiation might be the hardest part. What's hardest for one person may not be the hardest for someone else.

Chapter 3:

The Side Effects

Chemo Brain

One of the biggest things that happened to me when I was going through chemo was what is known as "chemo brain," a common term used to describe thinking and memory problems that can occur during and after cancer treatment. Anyone who's had children will know it well because it's very similar to "mom brain." I would walk into a room and forget why I was there. I would go home after chemo and would be talking to someone on the phone when I'd say, "I have to get off the phone right now. I can't talk anymore." My words and my thoughts would get jumbled, and I'd have difficulty putting sentences together.

Or sometimes I would be driving, and I would get discombobulated. Usually, we drive on autopilot from memory. But the chemo meant that sometimes I would be driving – especially at night when it was dark out

– and I wouldn't know where I was. I couldn't see buildings, I could only see lights, so I would be stopped at a red light and think, *I don't know where I'm going right now. I don't know which way to turn.* So I would have to slow down, physically look at street signs, and recheck every time I stopped the car. I didn't realize how bad nighttime driving was for me until it simply became more than I could manage. Eventually, my husband would drive me around.

I lost cognitive function and had a hard time explaining myself. I would be having a long, drawn-out conversation, get confused, and not know what I was going to say. That was really hard. Chemo, in general, is hard, but chemo brain was particularly hard because I felt like I was losing my brain a little bit too. Those types of things happen to a lot of people when they're going through chemo. At some point I had to stop worrying about social graces.

I had known at the time that there were free workshops and psychological services available through the Cross Cancer Institute to help improve my cognitive function. These were available to me and my loved ones for the rest of my life. I didn't take advantage of them in the beginning, but I wish I had. I thought I had everything under control and didn't need to go because I wasn't "crazy." I realize now what incredible opportunities I had and still have before me. Seeing a psychologist can be very expensive, but I've been offered the chance to see specialized psychologists who work with cancer patients for free. Two years after my diagnosis, I did take advantage of that service, as did my husband. He was able to go and talk about how it feels to be a caregiver and how to not only deal with his wife having cancer but later his mother. Classes are also available to children dealing with a parent having cancer, who in some cases lose that parent.

Looking back now, I don't think therapy should be an optional service; it should be mandatory for every cancer patient. I've received some very valuable coping tools through those services, which I'll write more about throughout this book. My advice to new cancer patients is not to let any stigma around mental health, asking for help, or taking medication get in the way of your recovery. There are tools to help you. It's a whole different game when you've got cancer. You may think you have everything under control, but sooner or later you will likely find out that you don't.

My Hair

I was told I would probably lose my hair starting around day fifteen of my twenty-one-day chemotherapy cycle. I had long hair when I got diagnosed; I had been growing it out. I joked that my goal was to be a mermaid so that I didn't have to wear a shirt anymore; I could just have my hair covering my chest. I had gotten to that point just when I got diagnosed with cancer. It was a bit sad to lose what I had worked so hard to grow, but the loss of my hair wasn't otherwise traumatic for me.

I cut my hair to shoulder length right after the diagnosis and cut bangs. I came home, and my daughter said, "Mom, your hair is ugly."

I said, "How do you know that hair is a trophy at the age of two-and-a-half?" *Thank you, Disney.*

It was probably day fifteen or sixteen after chemo had started when I put my hands through my hair and about ten hairs fell out in my hand. As I noted earlier, I knew something weird was happening because my head was starting to hurt. I thought to myself, *Okay. I can't control the fact that my hair is going to fall out, but I can control when it's going to fall out.* As I mentioned earlier, I've always liked having control of my life. I realized that I could let the situation control me, or I could do what I love and take control myself. I decided I was not going to sit and watch it fall out and be devastated by it.

So, I went to see my friend Chantal. She was my hairstylist and one of my best friends, who had been doing my hair for decades. I told her she needed to shave my head. She washed my hair and cut it with scissors first. Then she took a straight razor to it and shaved it right down to the wood for me. It felt like I was getting a new hairdo that day. I never felt like I was losing my hair to cancer. I thought, *Look at me. I'm hardcore. I have a shaved head!*

I went home the night that I shaved my head and took a photo of myself. I posted it on Facebook with the caption, "Hey, I shaved my head. Not a bad bean. My head's cute," and just kind of put it out there.

My brother came to visit me a couple of days later and said, "You're so brave. I don't think I'd be able to put a picture of myself online after I just shaved my head."

I said, "I'm not that brave. I just thought that's what people would do."

"No," he said. "That's not just what people do, and I think that what you're doing is a really good thing for other people that have cancer." It would have felt more depressing to me if I had gotten my head shaved at the cancer wig center. I am glad I went to my hairstylist.

I had been advised to go to a place called Wig on 123rd Street. A lot of times, depending on your coverage, healthcare will cover the cost of a wig. Those ladies know everything there is to know about wigs. I walked in, and there were what I call "old lady wigs" everywhere. They had every style, every color. I tried on so many short hairdo ones and thought, *This is not me. No.* Then I started trying on longer ones. I said, "If I'm going to wear a wig, I'm going to wear a kick-ass long wig where I feel super awesome." So, I got a wig that was similar to my hair before I cut it, but not exactly the same. I had to laugh at that experience because not only did I choose this awesome wig, the color I had chosen was called Rocky Road. A sign of things to come perhaps?

I also had to get the wig altered. Altered? Yes, I apparently have a very small head, so the ladies at Wig had to sew the inside to make it fit my wee little head. Wigs are not all one-size-fits-all.

I took really good care of my wig. The one thing I would recommend is to get synthetic hair. I didn't have time to be doing my hair, if I had a wig. A wig made with human hair still has to be made up; it acts like real hair. Whereas, with a synthetic wig, it's like Barbie hair. You just stick it in a bowl of cold water with some shampoo, rinse it out, put it on the showerhead to dry, and the style is already there. For me, that was a lot easier. On top of that, synthetic hair is less expensive than real hair.

It was recommended to me that I get somebody who knows how to cut synthetic hair to make it look less like a wig. So, I took it to a drag queen, who is also a hairstylist, and he did an incredible job of cutting it to give it less of a wig feel. He told me to use a lot of hairspray in it so that it didn't look so new. He taught me how to wash it and the right type of brush to use. I received so many great tips there, and it was a really good experience. I was trying to embrace all these new experiences, even if I hadn't asked for them. It's fun trying on wigs!

Most of the time, however, I didn't wear my wig. It was hot and very uncomfortable, and I would get what felt like hot flashes when I was wearing it. I wore my wig when I didn't want people to notice I had cancer—for work or occasions when I didn't feel like talking about the fact that I had cancer, didn't want to stand out, or be noticed. Many people didn't know I had cancer because when I was working, it was an appointment to support other people to look and feel their best. They were the focus, not me. The rest of the time, I would wear slouchy toques (a beanie or knitted hat for you Americans), a scarf, or a hat. But most of the time, I rocked my beautiful bald head. After all, I had a tiny, cute little bean of a head; I might as well embrace it.

By the way, being bald is very cold. I had to wear a hoodie with the hood up when I went to bed, so I didn't freeze all night. Sometimes I would wear a toque to bed, but a hoodie was better because it covered my neck. I finally understood the meaning of a nightcap.

When I got cancer, people I didn't even know came out of the woodwork. An acquaintance of mine was a make-up artist. She contacted me during treatment and said, "My friend Natasha is a photographer, and she and I want to do something nice for you. We're coming to your house to do your make-up and take photos of you. We'll do a little photo shoot of you in treatment."

I thought, *Yeah. Let's do it*. Any distraction during cancer treatment is welcome. It made me feel like I didn't have cancer. They came to my house and made me feel pretty and normal. They took pictures of me and my wig. They took pictures of me bald. They took pictures of me with my kids. I look at those photos now, and I think how important it is that people see how beautiful you can feel as a bald person and how important it is to document your time with the disease. My kids are so little in those photos, and it reminds me how amazing they were through the whole process.

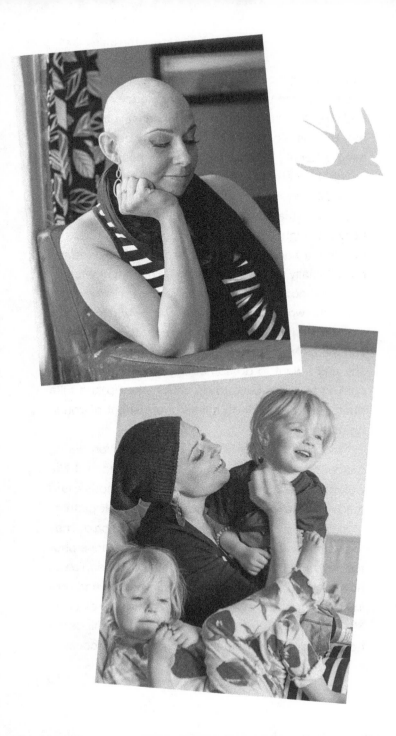

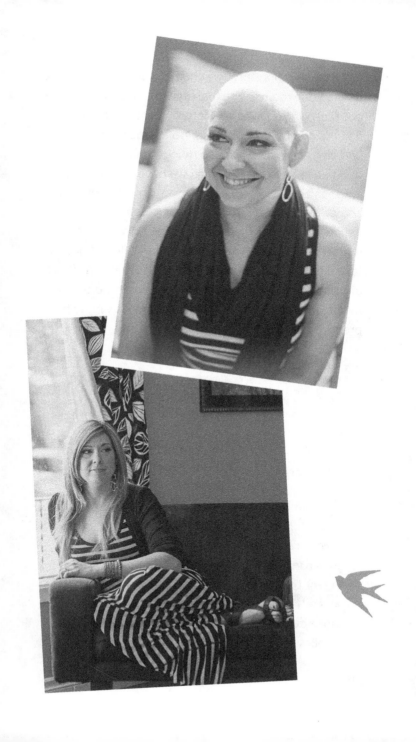

To those going through chemo, your hair does not define you. You're more than just your hair. I would go out feeling like I was rocking my bald head, and the first thing people would do is look at me with sad eyes and say, "Hey, how are you doing?" Just because we don't have hair doesn't mean we have to look sick. To emphasize this, I would draw on my eyebrows, put some lipstick on, and put some blush on. I wore a headscarf or a big, slouchy toque. I'd wear big earrings. I kept a sense of normalcy in my life. I'd get up, take a shower, get dressed, and put on makeup. There are days I wouldn't feel like it, but when I did those things, I would feel better. It wasn't about trying to look pretty, it was about trying to feel normal.

NEW PERSPECTIVE: FROM HAIR STYLIST CHANTAL GIRARD

I was in the basement of my house doing laundry when I received a phone call from Kristi. She told me she had felt a lump one day when she was in the kitchen. Then she told me she had stage three breast cancer, and I was in shock. She was so strong and confident on the phone. When I went to her house to visit a few days later, she was sitting on her bed, and we discussed it in more detail. I remember telling her she would be okay, even though in my heart I wasn't sure.

I knew the only things she needed to hear were positive, kind, and loving words.

Throughout her journey, I was very scared and worried about her, but I never showed it. I knew I needed to be strong to support her and just show her love. One of the hardest things I had to do was shave her head. Everything inside of me was crumbling, and I felt devastated for my young friend fighting this terrible disease. On the outside, however, I was happy and strong and encouraging. It took every ounce of courage and strength for me not to burst into tears in those moments. I held it together for her. When she left the salon, I allowed myself to cry for my friend that I loved.

Exhaustion

Between days ten and fourteen of a chemo cycle, my energy was really compromised. Chemo and radiation are cumulative, so the more chemo I had, the bigger my side effects became. The last month of chemo was when I felt the worst. I wasn't going out in public, I wasn't at the mall, and I didn't go to work. I even skipped Easter dinner at my in-laws the first month of treatment because I didn't know what to expect. But after four or five months, I thought, *It doesn't matter, I'm going to the mall.* I wasn't going to let it disrupt or interfere with my life more than it already had.

Eyebrows and Eyelashes

The last month of chemo was when I lost my eyebrows and eyelashes. *Really? I'm on the last one! I had them all the way until now*! They were the part of me that made me not feel sick. Nothing made me look sicker than not having eyebrows. After that, drawing on my eyebrows became very important.

The Cross was the place I felt the most normal when I had cancer because everyone was bald there. No one was looking at me with sympathetic eyes because what I was going through was just everyday there. Fortunately, they also have a program called "Look Good, Feel Good." They teach patients how to draw on eyebrows and the best kinds of creams and makeups to use for people going through cancer.

I took the class, and that helped me feel a little more normal. It wasn't about feeling like a fashion model; it was about not wanting to look sick. I think that looking sick is what makes cancer patients not feel so great about themselves; it's also what attracts potentially unwelcome attention. Men can get away with being bald, but if a woman is bald, people think, *Oh, she's got cancer. She's sick*. That's a discussion that I feel needs to change.

Toenails and Fingernails

During the last couple of months of chemo, my hands and feet really hurt. I couldn't wear high heels, because

I couldn't figure out where my foot was landing. I couldn't feel my foot. It was a bizarre side effect of the treatment.

That's when I lost my toenails and my fingernails as well. The nails that didn't fall out, fell to pieces. My nails became very flimsy, and I still have lasting effects from the chemo. Eight years later, my toes and my fingers still feel numb. Nerve damage occurred, so I don't have the feeling I used to have pre-diagnosis.

All of these side effects have been challenging to overcome. But I always say now, "It is what it is." I can't control the fact that I have them. Cancer was an invitation for me to surrender my pre-diagnosis control issues and just accept what is. Before, I would have asked myself, *How can I fix this?* Now, I just get a manicure.

Chapter 4:

Chemo, Kids, and Loneliness

One of the saddest parts about having cancer was that my kids weren't allowed into my bedroom because I was too sick and immunocompromised to have kids and germs in my room. A lot of times I would hear them just outside my door, crying for me, and I couldn't help them. My immune system was also compromised, so I had to be careful.

I remember one time when my son Noah slid his teddy bear under my door and was calling me, "Mummy, Mummy, Mummy." My heart ached. They were around for it all; they just didn't see me sick all the time. They could come into my room and visit me on occasion, but since they were two-and-a-half, they wanted to be all over me. If I'd just had surgery, or if I was in chemo, it was very uncomfortable to have them on top of me. But I never got frustrated with them. I am proud to say I never redirected my anger at them.

"Mom guilt" came into effect a lot. *I should be being their mom right now. They need me and here I am sitting in bed doing nothing*, I'd think. But I was healing, trying to take care of myself. As a people-pleaser and a giver, the worst thing in the world was making other people sad. It made me very upset that I had to sit there while my kids were missing me.

I feel like I lost a lot of time with them as babies. It was a formative time for them when it was important to hold them and make them feel better, but instead, I had to hold myself and make myself feel better. As a mother, that was really hard, but I felt like I didn't have a choice. I had to do it, to be around for my kids in the long run.

So, I lost myself in books and TV and tried not to think about the fact that I might not be there for my kids someday. Instead, I fought hard to be there for them, and I was there for them as much as I could be. Even when I had a nanny and had friends coming over to help, I would still get up and play when them, talk to them, and take them to the park if I felt well enough.

I had tried to prepare my kids for what was to come after I got the diagnosis. I sat down with them and said I was sick. Since they were so young, they didn't understand what "sick" really meant. I said, "You know when you have a cold, you guys have a runny nose and don't feel very well? Mommy is like that, except instead of a runny nose, I am going to lose my hair." Losing my hair was the only symptom I could think of that I thought they would understand.

So they didn't notice really that I was sick until I came home with my shaved head. Both of them were very funny about that. I took off my toque and they said, "Your hair is pokey, Mom." They just wanted to touch my head.

I said, "I'll be able to wear fun hats now." But they really didn't understand.

When they got a little bit older, I used a technique I learned from a therapist. I told them, "When you have small sick, like a runny nose or a fever, we give you small medicine, and you go to a regular doctor. But Mommy has big sick, so we have to use big medicine, and I have to go to a special hospital with special doctors. Sometimes the big medicine doesn't work, but most of the time it does. And right now, it's working for Mommy."

I never used the word cancer, because it wasn't useful at that point. They were too little to understand what cancer is. They were at an age when they still thought eating crayons was an acceptable thing. So my intention was just to keep my language simple. I told them there were going to be some changes going on, such as having Grandma and Grandpa around a lot more. They were going to have a nanny taking care of them. They were so little, I don't think they even caught on to what I was communicating. Toddlers are little narcissists, so they were probably like, *Yeah, but can you turn Dora on?* But they were excited to see Grandma and Grandpa every other weekend.

One day when my daughter was in first grade, she came home from school and said, "Mom, we learned about Terry Fox today. He had cancer."

I said, "Oh, yeah? What did you learn?" I was terrified that she was going to put two and two together now she'd heard the word "cancer," but I wasn't sure if she knew that's what I had.

She replied, "He ran across the whole country. And then his cancer came back and his leg got sick."

I said, "Yeah?"

And she continued, "And then he turned into a statue."

That's when I started talking to her about it. I said, "That's what I had. Mommy had cancer." By the time they reached first grade, my kids participated in the Terry Fox run, an annual, non-competitive charity event to raise money for cancer research. I came to school one day, and my daughter had a t-shirt on that said, "I'm running for my mom." That was the first time I realized my kids knew what cancer was.

Although I did not give much thought to my mortality as I underwent cancer treatment, I did meet other women going through breast cancer who passed away. One of those women had children the same age as mine, which made me think about what would happen to my kids if I died. The thought of it made me sad, but I was confident that I had a good family support system. They would still have their dad, their grandparents, and a strong extended family on both sides.

I also witnessed the support that came from the community for the families of other women who did not make it. Of course, the role of a mother can never be completely replaced, but people do come in to take over the jobs of a mother. I knew my kids would be well taken care of by my family, friends, and even women I met through therapy groups.

I often got asked, "How are your kids doing with everything?"

I'd reply, "They're two-and-a-half years old, so they still yell at me for milk, they still want me to bring them Cheerios, and they still ask me to play with them." Nothing really changed for them; it was me who felt bad that I couldn't be there more for them.

Older kids need a lot more support if their parent is going through cancer, especially psychologically, because they understand what's going on. For many kids in Canada, their first exposure to the idea of cancer is through learning about Terry Fox, and he died. But that's not always what happens. If my kids had been older when I was diagnosed, I would have told them, "I'm not a statistic. We don't know what's going to happen. Nobody knows the future. Many people survive cancer. No one goes through life unscathed. We're just going to take it one day at a time."

Loneliness

I spent so much time alone in my room that I had to look for diversions. Right outside my window was a giant tree. While I watched TV, that tree would keep me company. I watched the squirrels play in the tree. I didn't go so far as to sit and talk to the tree, but

I would think, *It's just you and me here.* I had a friend that later pointed out that we can't be alone when we're in nature because everything around us is alive. That made me realize I should have been outside more when I was sick; I think it would have helped me to be in my garden and get my hands in the dirt.

As I was in bed, I would sit and think about being alone and how I was sick and tired of being sick and tired. I was tired of listening to my kids outside the door being sad. And then all of these feelings came up like, *I'm sick and my kids are out there. I don't have time to have breast cancer, I have to take care of my kids.* I worried I was going to lose my job. Toxic and illogical thoughts came about my husband not doing enough, or my friends not doing enough, just because I was by myself all day. Then I would be worried all day long about getting sicker. I had to take my temperature frequently because if I had a temperature over 38 degrees Celsius (100.4 degrees Fahrenheit), I was supposed to go to the emergency room. I had a lot of bone pain, and I couldn't get up.

Thank God for George R.R. Martin, because I read *Game of Thrones* for six months straight. It was one thing that kept my brain occupied. Despite reading a lot and watching a lot of TV, there were times I wanted to sleep but couldn't because I was so worried about dying. Or I would obsesses about my symptoms, *I feel like I should be more nauseated. That's supposed to be a symptom. How come I'm not more nauseated?* As if I were doing cancer wrong or something.

As a reminder, there is no right way to have cancer. To get myself out of these funks, I would leave the house. I would get out of bed, take a shower, and put on real clothes (not just pajamas and leisurewear). Something about leaving my house, even if it was to take a small walk around the block, helped to tame my irrational and uncensored thoughts. I suppose it was my way of staying in the moment. Anxiety can take hold of you when you're stuck in your bedroom being sick. When I would get outside and walk or get in my car to get a Chai Tea Latte at Starbucks, it made me realize I could still take small actions to make myself feel better. Being mindful and relaxing the brain is hard when existential anxiety is top-of-mind, but when it's possible to do it, it helps.

Chapter 5:

Support Systems

When it comes to support, step one is figuring out what you need, and the next step is asking for what you need. Some people want to be left alone; they don't want people to see them sick. Some people want somebody to make them lunch one day. Others want company to watch TV with them the whole time they are sick. Some people want someone to hold their hair back while they're throwing up.

For me, it wasn't until after I was done with my chemo treatments that I realized I needed somebody to be there for me mentally, someone to hold my hand the whole time because I was really lonely. Thankfully, I did have several support systems available to me. One tool helped me, and I learned later in therapy it's called the "Ring Theory." It was developed by psychologist Susan Silk and her friend Barry Goldman, and it's a valuable approach to supporting people.

Here's how it works.

1. Draw a circle. In the circle, write the name of the person experiencing the traumatic event.
2. Draw a larger circle around the first one. In this circle, write the name of the person closest to the crisis the person in the center of the ring is experiencing.
3. Continue drawing circles around each prior circle, and writing the names of the people next closest to the person in the center of the ring.

Parents and children come before more distant relatives. Intimate friends come closer to the center, and less intimate friends go in the larger circles.

Here are the rules of Ring Theory. The person in the center of the ring can say anything he or she wants to, to anyone, anywhere. Therefore, I could complain and whine and say things such as, "Why me?" or "Life is unfair!" Everyone else can say those things too, but only to people in the larger rings, never to me.

When talking to a person in a ring smaller than yours, the goal is to help that person. Listening is often more helpful than talking, but if you're going to talk, first ask yourself if what you are going to say is likely to provide comfort and support. If not, don't say it. Never give advice. People suffering from trauma don't need advice, they need love, comfort, and support.

For example you could say, "I'm sorry," "This must be really hard for you," or "Can I bring you Mexican lasagna?" But don't say, "You should hear what happened to my uncle who had cancer," "This is what you should do," or "This makes me so sad." If you want to cry or complain, do it with someone in an outer ring. In other words, "comfort" goes into the ring, and "dumping" goes out.

To use a personal example, if I'm in the inner circle and you are a casual friend who comes to visit me and my hair loss is making you uncomfortable, you have to go outside the circle before you talk about it. You can only talk about it with someone in a larger circle than yours, which is not my husband or my family.

THE RING THEORY

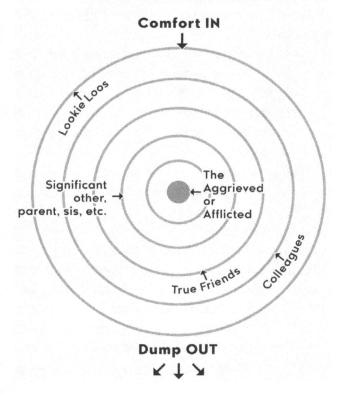

Comfort IN

Lookie Loos

Significant other, parent, sis, etc. →

The Aggrieved or Afflicted

True Friends

Colleagues

Dump OUT

The Role of Family

On the recommendation of a friend, I read *Crazy Sexy Cancer* by Kris Carr when I first got sick. One of the things I took from that book was that cancer has a weird power over people. People think if they say the word "cancer," they are going to get the disease or make it worse. People whisper about it, and whispering gives cancer power. My dad and my mom started to do that around me. Talking about cancer openly and squarely made me feel like it's not that powerful. It was like saying, "You're not that big of a deal, cancer."

There is a whole marketing machine around cancer on TV, in movies and commercials. All we hear is it's going to kill you. And what I read from Kris Carr was, "No. You can do this." That book helped me think about cancer differently. Don't think about it as you've been told to think about it.

I made my dad stand in the kitchen with me one day, and I told him, "I need you to say the word cancer. Say, 'Kristi, you have cancer.'"

My dad said quietly, "Kristi, you have cancer."

I said, "No, you need to say it loudly."

I told my family at the beginning, "I don't want you all standing around feeling sorry for me and looking sad and forlorn. I'm already feeling shitty. I don't want to have to support you in the midst of supporting myself."

So, my family and friends were very good about keeping me afloat, even if they felt sad. That was another thing that was not my job, managing their feelings about my cancer. It was their responsibility to 'dump out' and manage their own reactions to my situation. My mom would come every other weekend and take care of me. I know she was very sad and had a hard time with it, but she never once let me see it. I was clear about the fact that I didn't want a bunch of pity. I said, "This is my story. This is what's happening to me. I want to deal with it. I don't want you to have to be worried about it too."

So, we would joke around with each other and use humor to get through it. When my family would be over, for example, I might use my cancer to get out of household chores, "I can't do the dishes; I've got cancer." The lighter mood helped us all. Making light of my cancer was another way of making me feel like cancer is not that powerful.

Friends to the Rescue

There were friends that stepped in and helped me in a variety of ways. They brought me Dairy Queen. They would come to visit and keep me company. Sometimes I just wanted someone to hang out with during the day. Lying in bed day in and day out is a lonely, lonely thing. Having a friend to watch Downton Abbey with for an hour meant the world to me.

I also had a long-standing friendship with Wendy, a woman I had met when I was eighteen. She came to a lot of my treatments. She even invited me to her house when I was so sick that I didn't want my kids to see me. She would make me breakfast and take care of me. She'd make me a cinnamon bun or soup, filling the role of mother for me when my mom wasn't able to be there.

Interestingly, the friends I thought were going to be there for me were not necessarily the ones there for me. And the friends that I thought weren't going to show up for me were sometimes the ones who were at my house every day, changing poopy diapers and putting my babies to bed at night for me. That was eye-opening.

But I couldn't get mad at the friends that didn't show up because everyone deals with cancer in a different way. Whoever wanted to help could help, and whoever couldn't deal with it, couldn't deal with it. I had one friend that said, "I can't talk to you because my dad died of cancer. We can't talk about it." I had to accept that was their issue, not mine, and let it go.

Scheduling Support

After getting diagnosed, I had a whole slew of people come to me and say, "Whatever I can do for you, just let me know." If you get sick and people make that offer, take down their names. Take their phone numbers. You might not want their help at the time, but you will need them later on in some capacity, perhaps to buy groceries or give you a ride to chemo. If you need a sandwich made for you or somebody to keep you company, call them. They might not have time the day you call them, but they may another day. In the meantime, call somebody else.

I had so many people bring me food, a lot of which was lasagna. Many people have to take a break from lasagna after cancer, including seafood lasagna. I would put it in the freezer and maybe never eat it, depending on how nauseated I was feeling. But at least they brought it. It felt like they did something for me, and that's all they could do. So I was grateful for the people who showed up in whatever capacity they could.

Most people don't know how to help, so telling them what you need keeps them from having to figure out ways to support you. I remember sending out emails that said, "Hey, everyone, I'm doing okay, but my husband is struggling with meals. We need some help." And people would come help.

Or I'd post something on Facebook. Not everyone wants to announce on Facebook that they're sick, but it can be efficient when you need something. I didn't use it to inform people all the time of how I was doing. Again, that wasn't my job. My job was to get better, and sometimes that meant asking for help. There are also several apps and websites that can help schedule "meal trains" where people sign up to provide meals on certain days. Another idea is to find a volunteer "advocate," someone to act as the point of contact for managing your schedule of needs or updates on your health.

Now, when someone I know gets sick, I know what to say. I say, "I'm here to support you. What do you need? If you don't know what you need, here is my phone number. Call me when you do."

Child Support

We had a nanny even before I got diagnosed, and she helped just by being there during the day for the kids when I was sick. A month after I got diagnosed, she quit. She thought she was just coming to look after some twins, right? She didn't take the job to become a mom. So we hired another nanny who stepped in and was very helpful.

I was very privileged to be able to have a nanny who could take care of my kids every day. I had a good daycare I could take them to as well. And my parents came every other weekend for six months to take care of the twins, drive them wherever they needed to go, and take care of me. I had a friend who lived next door who let my parents stay there every two weeks. She said, "We are here for whatever you need. Your parents can be here whenever they want." That was so helpful.

Support doesn't have to look a certain way. People might have a preconceived idea of what supporting a person with cancer looks like, but it can be as simple as offering space for your caregivers to come and stay.

It can be lasagna. It can be coming in to look after children. I had a lady I didn't even know come to my house with groceries. She was a friend of someone I used to work with who had heard about my situation. She said, "I can't cook, but I can buy groceries."

One mistake I made was asking for help too late in the process, especially with my husband. I didn't know to tell him how I needed to be helped. At the beginning of my diagnosis, he had said he was going to be around all the time and was going to take time off from work. In reality, that couldn't happen. He's a business owner, and we still needed to pay the bills. But that was a disappointment for me. My expectation was A, and I got B. He also thought that since we had a nanny at the time, the nanny would take care of me. But, no, the nanny was taking care of our kids.

We also had two specific people that would come Wednesday and Friday evenings to help us out with the kids after our nanny had left. On Wednesdays, it was a friend that I never thought would want to be there. But when I got sick, she immediately asked, "What can I do? Can I come over? Can I change your babies' diapers? I'm going to feed them." And she would read them bedtime stories and put them to bed. On Fridays, one of my husband's high school friends would come over and put the kids to bed. He took videos of our kids going to sleep and sent them to me. It was so sweet. So again, bottom line, the people that were consistently there for us were not necessarily the ones we expected.

Chemo Buddy

While I was going through chemo treatment, I would often see the same people. Over time we'd get to know each other. Each of us would bond with a particular person, who would informally become our "chemo buddy." When I met my chemo buddy Jen, it was such a relief. We are the same age, her kids are just a little bit older than mine, and our husbands have similar personalities. We would even both wear the same cute outfits to chemo, which is why we noticed one another in the first place. When we finally sat beside each other, I had someone to talk to who was going through basically the same experiences, and I felt like I wasn't alone anymore. Having a chemo buddy was helpful because she knew that there were things I wouldn't want to hear. For example, for a lot of people going through cancer, being told to stay positive every day is not helpful. It's a canned response that I didn't have to worry about hearing from her.

JULIE'S GUIDE FOR THINGS YOU SHOULDN'T SAY OR DO TO PEOPLE WITH CANCER

You would have loved my friend Julie. She was the best. She made me laugh every day. She was funny and irreverent,

and I miss her a lot. Many of these tips are from her. I know she would love me sharing them with you.

1. When somebody tells you they have cancer, don't tell them about your aunt or your uncle or your cousin that passed away from cancer.

2. I got told I was lucky. "You're lucky this is breast cancer. Breast cancer is one of the best kinds of cancer you can get." It's still cancer. Please don't tell someone with cancer that they are lucky.

3. I was also told, "This must have brought you and your husband closer together." I replied, "Are you kidding me? We hate each other right now. I'm not happy with him, and he's not happy with me." Having cancer puts marriages in a very stressful situation.

4. Don't create drama or express pity. Someone asked me once, "Was the cancer in your lymph nodes?" When I answered that it was, they looked at me with pity. But that was my reality. It was in my lymph nodes. I was just answering their question, not looking for pity.

5. "Stay strong; stay positive." Those are not helpful things for a cancer patient to hear because they're already fighting for their life. Of course, they're strong, and, of course, they're trying to be positive. But you have to allow them to have space to be sad and feel depressed.

Maybe it's not okay to be like that every day, but staying strong and positive all the time is a tall order, especially when the most horrific thing is happening to you.

6. Don't just check-in and then leave as soon as you have concluded that everything is fine. Regardless of what the person with cancer says, everything is not okay.

7. Don't completely avoid people with cancer. I was surprised by how many people thought they could catch cancer from me. Maybe they worried that I'd break down and start bawling my eyes out, but it sucks being treated like a leper.

8. People on social media would say things like, "Kristi, you're my hero. You're so strong." Some days I felt like being somebody's hero was a burden. I just couldn't be doing everything all the time. Plus, they didn't really know what was going on. They would read what I was sharing publicly, without realizing what I was dealing with on the inside. That's why I've always appreciated my family and my group of friends.

Chapter 6:

Mastectomy, Menopause, and More

Most commonly, if a breast cancer patient is going to have a mastectomy and chemotherapy, she is given the mastectomy first, then chemotherapy, and then she might have radiation. But because my cancer was so far advanced, I had to have chemotherapy first to shrink everything, and then I would have the mastectomy followed by radiation.

Ironically, as I prepared for surgery, I was more worried about missing work, the people I had yet to tell about my cancer, and how my kids were going to handle my recovery than I was about how I was going to handle the surgery. I didn't think about the possibility of dying; fatalistic thoughts would have consumed me if I had let them. I already felt like I was at the bottom of a mountain there was no way I could climb; I just had to focus on getting through each step.

When I first went to meet with my general surgeon, before I even met with my oncologist, she asked if I had thought about having a bilateral mastectomy, which means both breasts removed. I said, "Yeah, that's what I want." I thought that it would always be in the back of my head that my other breast could get cancer.

She replied, "Okay, good."

Now that I've been through cancer, I know from other women I've met in support groups and other surgeons I've talked to that doctors are not supposed to suggest bilateral mastectomies to just anybody. Unless someone has had genetic testing done and they have the genetic type of cancer, it is not recommended that they have a healthy breast removed. Getting cancer in the opposite breast is like getting cancer in your foot or your lungs or your liver. It's a different part of your body; they're not connected except by genetics.

Perhaps it was because I was very young to have breast cancer, but the plastic surgeon agreed with the general surgeon that it was better for me to have both breasts removed. At that point, there was so much information coming at me that I trusted the surgeons I was working with to make the right decision for me. I first thought that the reconstruction would be done at the same time as the mastectomy, but for me, that wasn't an option because I had to have radiation after the mastectomy. Radiation and reconstruction can't happen at the same time, so I had to wait at least a whole year before starting the reconstruction process.

Because I was having both of my breasts removed, two types of surgeries were available. One is where they do a tummy tuck. They take the skin and fat from your lower abdomen along with your blood and muscles so that things start to grow and adhere in the new location. That's the limousine of breast reconstruction because you're getting a tummy tuck and new boobs!

But for me, I didn't have enough tissue in my abdomen to have that surgery. I had to have what's called latissimus dorsi reconstruction. This is where they take the large, flat muscle on the back that stretches to the sides. With this surgery, I had to have incisions on my front side and backside, which required a healing period of eight to twelve weeks. It's a heavy-duty surgery. Everything I read about the surgery was horrific. I was terrified I'd look crazy and deformed. I looked up photos on the internet, which is always a mistake, and saw scars that were scary and big.

That made me question, *Do I need breasts that bad? Do I need to have two boobs?* I questioned if I should just have both boobs removed, to be symmetrical, and leave it at that. But in the end, I told myself, *I can do this. I do want to be symmetrical and I want both breasts.*

Despite my confidence in my decision, I felt like I was losing part of my femininity by losing my breasts. It felt like I was going to lose part of myself mentally with the loss of my physical breasts. I worried about my sex life because it was highly interactive with my breasts. I wondered if that would change, or if I'd even be able to have any feeling where my breasts had been. Would my husband even still find me attractive? We'd had talks about it, and I asked him, "Do you care that I won't have breasts?"

He said, "You have to do whatever it is that you need to do to get through this." That made me feel confident that he wasn't going anywhere after the surgery. He loved me no matter what, and it didn't matter what I looked like.

With my mastectomy, they gave me a surgery date. I was supposed to get both of my breasts removed at the same time. But at the eleventh hour I decided I only wanted my left breast off at that time, which was the cancerous side, and I was going to leave my right side until I could have reconstruction. Then, I'd get the plastic surgeon to take that one off, and he could rebuild both breasts at the same time. In retrospect, I should have gotten them both off at the same time because I had to live with one breast for two years. There was a huge waiting list. I was what was called a "singleton," or a person living with one boob.

In Canada's public healthcare, the cost of the surgery is covered. If I would have chosen to pay to get an augmentation done, I could have gotten new breasts right away, but it's a very expensive surgery. Because I waited for public health, it was two years between the time that I lost my first breast and the time I got my second breast removed and had reconstruction. There was a huge line of people waiting to get breast reconstruction done, and the surgeon that I chose is very popular. But I'm really glad I waited for him.

The day before surgery I thought, *I'm getting amputated tomorrow. Oh my god, this is major surgery*. But at the hospital, it was just another routine day surgery. A general surgeon operated on me; she gave me what's called a radical mastectomy. They took out fourteen lymph nodes and three were positive for cancer. It had started to move into my lymphatic system, but it hadn't vascularized, so it hadn't grown legs and moved through my body. On my left side, I was just left with skin and ribs, not even a nipple. There was nothing left of my breast, just a scar.

I had been really afraid that I wouldn't feel like myself when I woke up. I woke up with my husband and my best friend by my side. They were being especially supportive and adoring and I was being well taken care of, but I remember thinking to myself, *I just want my mom here. I love you both, but I just want my mom.*

I looked down to see I had been put into this pretty blue, flowered, stretchy tube top. Of course, it was not what I was expecting. Hospital wear is typically bunk. I put my hand down to my chest to see if I still had feeling there. I was numb from the drugs, but I still felt like myself, which was a huge relief to me. Even though I didn't have a breast there anymore, I still had some feeling. It wasn't just a big empty space.

The resident nurses came in quite early to look at the surgery site and how I was healing. I was terrified to look at myself. I told them not to take the bandage off yet, but it was too late. The tube top and my bandages came off quickly. I had a voice inside my head saying, *You can do it!* I looked down. I saw a line of stitches that went from my sternum straight across my chest and ended under my arm. It was red and swollen, but it was amazing. My surgeon had done a remarkable job.

I had been given something called a "block" when they gave me the anesthetic. It lasted an extremely long time, so I didn't have a lot of pain with the surgery. Still, seven years later there are parts of my underarms and my breasts that I can't feel. That's part of my "new normal."

After that, the nurses said, "Alright, you're all done. You can go home."

I was like, "You just took off my breast! Don't I have to stay here for a couple of days?"

They said, "Nope, you're ready to go home. Bye!"

I realized that every time I went to the Cross, what felt like a life or death situation for me and brought up all of these emotions was just another day on the job for them. This is what they did all day long. That's what helped me shift my mindset to, *My job is to get better.*

In the weeks after the surgery, I felt invincible. I thought, *Look at me go. I'm surviving!* I didn't feel ugly. I felt like I looked okay. After working in fashion and seeing people struggle with their body image for so long, I had come to realize that most people don't notice what we think is "wrong" with ourselves. I knew I could camouflage my chest so that no one would even know I only had one breast.

I wore baggy, flowy tops and usually a sports bra. Underwire bras would slide so that one side would be up by my ear and the other underneath my breast. I never wore a traditional prosthetic because they're heavy, lumpy, and uncomfortable. If I wanted to wear something more form-fitting, I used a piece that goes inside bathing suits. It was a contoured, light foam insert that, when I was wearing a triangle top, it looked like I had a breast. I bought mine at the bathing suit store. It was meant for small-chested women who could buy two. Nobody noticed I was wearing it. I was off-kilter when I was getting dressed, but I managed.

For those two years, I'd go to work with customers who would be complaining about their bodies in the changing rooms. I would hear, "Oh God, I don't like my thighs." Or, "I don't like my fat arms." Whatever it is, right?

I said, "We can camouflage anything. What do you notice about me?"

And they said, "Nothing."

And I said, "I have one breast." They said they never would have known. Bingo.

Even though it was an emotional journey for me to have the mastectomy, it was the easier part of my treatment compared to chemotherapy. The hard part of having chemo was being sick and being by myself so much. I got lonely and spent too much time in my head. It was also six months long, whereas with the mastectomy I was only in the hospital for one day.

I've known a lot of women, however, who struggled with their mastectomies. Some women can't even take their shirts off in front of their husbands. I had gone on the internet to look at what mastectomies look like, but the majority of photos I saw were from people complaining about how bad their surgeon was and how they had a terrible mastectomy. "This is what cancer did to my body," they'd say.

I didn't see one post that said, "Hey, look at my chest, it looks awesome!" And so, I decided to take a photo of myself and say, "Hey, this is what a mastectomy scar looks like." I'm proud of it. I don't think it looks horrific. I think I look pretty good. Don't be scared, was basically what I wanted to say. It's not the worst thing that can happen to you. And I had a really pretty nightgown on. It was very cathartic.

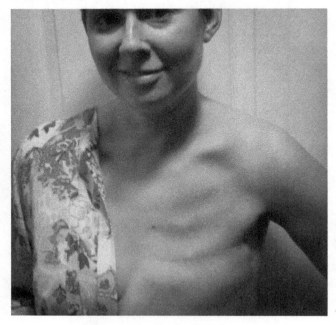

The reason that I did it, and why I'm telling this story, is for the women who can't even talk about their experience with breast cancer. I feel I need to be that voice for those women.

I know some women don't have a support system. They might have husbands that have feelings about their wives not having breasts anymore, or who don't know how to be supportive. For the women who hate their scars, *you will be okay*. Even though you've lost your breast, you're still you. You're more than your boobs, just like you're more than your hair. Whatever it is that makes you feel feminine can be replicated with enhancements.

I do recognize that for some women, breasts are a huge part of their sex lives. That can be extremely hard to adjust to. But you can figure out new ways to make yourself feel good. Have honest conversations with your partner and don't be afraid to ask hard questions and be okay with the answers. The truth is, a lot of marriages don't survive cancer. Yes, there's a breast cancer machine out there doing a lot of research, raising money, and so forth. But, the down and dirty of breast cancer is really sad. It's heartbreaking and emotional when couples can't make it through. My husband and I had our fair share of arguments throughout the treatment process. But in the end, the process is about you. Decisions that you make need to be based on how you feel about you.

Menopause at 37

After I was done with my first year of treatment, I was put on Tamoxifen. Tamoxifen is a drug that shuts estrogen production down, which is what fueled my estrogen-positive cancer.

An unexpected side effect was that I started going through menopause at the age of thirty-seven. I had hot flashes, night sweats, and my emotions were unpredictable. That was something I wasn't prepared for; I didn't think I'd have to navigate that as a young woman in my thirties.

I had to watch the fabrics I was wearing; anything man-made caused a hot flash. I would break out into a sweat if I had a hot tea in my hand. I had to change the sheets on my bed and pajamas to wicking fabrics, so I didn't wake up drenched in sweat every night. The list goes on and on, but the worst side effect was vaginal dryness; it hurt every time I'd have sex. I experienced one thing after another, and that was something I didn't know how to deal with. There are medications on the market that help with this side effect, but they all contained estrogen so I couldn't take them.

Post-menopause, my body has become more apple-shaped; I've gained weight in places I never did before. I can't just "work it off" because it's not something that can be worked off. And since I don't have estrogen, I'm losing my hair. I'm done with my child-rearing years, but going through menopause makes me feel older than I am. When I first realized I was going through it I thought, *Oh god, I'm like an old crone now. I've gone through that phase of my life!* It's hard, but it's yet another thing I accept that I don't have control over.

Since Tamoxifen shuts down all estrogen production in my body, sex isn't even on my radar. I don't feel like having it most days. I've stopped expecting to have the best time of my life during sex. I do try to enjoy the moment, but it's hard sometimes. I've had to try out different lubricants to make sure I'm using the right one. Some are extra drying, and some are moisturizing. I find that the more that I practice, the better sex feels, but if I leave it for too long, then it becomes painful again.

I wasn't even worried about my breasts anymore and whether they would change my sex life. I was more worried about having a non-existent sex life. It's hard to initiate sex when you have zero desire to do so and it feels like you're having sex with a cheese grater. Ouch. And that brings up feelings of guilt for not wanting sex as much as I used to, even though it's out of my control. They have some good programs at the Cross, including a new center called the Oasis Center where patients can go and talk about their sexual health. They share healthy ways to rejuvenate your sex life. Oncologists often bring it up as well. They'll say, "This is something that happens. We're here for you if you want to talk about it."

Lymphedema

I didn't realize I had lymphedema until about two years after I'd had my mastectomy, maybe even three. The word lymphedema comes from "lymphatic fluid." It is most commonly caused by the removal of lymph nodes as part of cancer treatment. It results from a blockage in the lymphatic system that prevents the lymphatic fluid from draining well. Thus, the fluid buildup results in swelling. All of a sudden, my left arm started to hurt, and I was having trouble getting it into my suit jackets.

I went to my doctor and was told I needed to have another appointment at the Cross. They have a great physiotherapy department there. I was measured and my left arm was found to be 15% bigger than my other arm. No wonder I was having difficulty getting it into blazers and long-sleeved shirts!

The only way to combat the condition is with compression therapy. I've had to come to terms with the fact that I have to wear a medical garment for the rest of my life on my left arm. Thankfully, I don't mind wearing it. The only time it's ever uncomfortable to talk about it is when somebody thinks I have a sports injury. They're not prepared for me to say, "No, I had breast cancer, and it's a symptom of a mastectomy." Even then, it's not uncomfortable for me; it's uncomfortable for the person who asked, who typically then regrets having asked such an unfortunate question.

Despite all of these changes in my body that were out of my control, I found some things I did have control over. For example, I may have to wear a compression sleeve on my arm for the rest of my life, but why not a cool one? I shop online and buy fun, patterned sleeves for people with lymphedema. I also started swimming; the pressure of the water moving over my arm makes me feel better. I might be bandaged, but I'm not broken.

Chapter 7:
Radiation

Not every breast cancer patient needs to have radiation. I asked my doctor, "Why do I need to have radiation? Didn't you guys get all the cancer when I had chemotherapy and when you took out the tumors and lymph nodes and calcifications?" I even had a radical mastectomy, which means they took everything out, the breast tissue, the skin, everything.

They said, "There's probably a 99% chance that all of the cancer was taken out of you, but there's a 1% chance that lying on the edge of a scar, some might be left. We want to make sure we got it all, and radiation takes care of that."

When I went to chemo, I didn't get the same nurses; they were different every time. With radiation, I was designated to one spot in the Cross. I had to go there every day, and I would see the same people. I had a radiation team.

It takes more time to park and get changed than it does to have radiation. It's so fast. The machines are incredibly precise. The first thing they did was measure the part of my body that was getting radiation because they wanted to make sure they didn't hit my heart or other internal organs.

At my very first treatment, they tattooed me with tiny dots on each side of my chest.

Then they had me line up exactly with the dots. A measurement tool came down on my chest but I wasn't lining up properly, so on my first day of scheduled radiation, I didn't get radiation. They told me, "The measurements are off. We have to recalibrate this whole machine, so you have to come back tomorrow." It was a relief because that made me feel like they were meticulously doing their job.

When I came back and the machine was properly calibrated, it was so loud that I didn't even know when I was getting radiation. The machine swung around me as I was on a table in an uncomfortable position. A weighted radiation blanket like the ones at the dentist lay on top of me and covered my body so the radiation didn't go onto a body part they didn't want to hit. I couldn't move because they especially didn't want the radiation to hit my heart or lungs.

I noticed that the room was bright and clinical. There was a light on the ceiling that shined down and had a ruler on it so they would know how to line me up. After the second radiation, I asked if they could dim the lights when I was getting radiation. I told myself it was kind of like a spa, just a horrible one. It made me feel more relaxed when the lights were dim.

My radiation burns weren't that bad. I basically felt like I had a bad sunburn. But to keep it real, I know people who have had radiation and got such severe burns, they had to go to emergency rooms or hospitals. My radiation burns just left pink skin on the left side of my body. It would be sensitive to touch, like a sunburn. But it did leave me permanently discolored on one side of my chest.

I had twenty treatments of radiation. I went every day for about a month, except on weekends. For me it was a breeze, but it made me feel beyond tired. The more treatments I had, the more tired I became. By the end, I was exhausted.

But I loved my team. Instead of going in and talking about radiation, we would have normal conversations about career, family, and our favourite TV shows. It was never about cancer, so that was refreshing. Since I saw them every day for twenty days, I got to know them. I've never been down there since. I am grateful I had them on my team, but I don't need to relive that time in my life.

Not So Fast

When the pathology for my mastectomy came and I got the results, it was the day before I was finishing radiation. A pathology is a report that comes back after a tumor is removed and sent to a lab for testing. There I was after nine months of cancer treatment, thinking

I was going to be done at the Cross. I was all ready to celebrate because my treatment was coming to an end. I beat cancer! Then my oncologist called me in and said, "We got the pathology back. Not only do you have estrogen receptor-positive cancer, but hormone receptor-positive cancer. This means you have to have one more year of treatment. It's not chemotherapy, but a drug called Herceptin."

I was devastated that I had not only one type of cancer, but two! The biopsy had been done in a different spot of my breast, so the second type of cancer was not initially caught. Instead of having one year of treatment, I would have over two years. I was disappointed and sad about the news, but I accepted it. I couldn't change the result; it was another thing I didn't have control over.

I've heard some breast cancer patients complain about their oncologists when getting that kind of news. But the way I looked at it was, hey, it's not a perfect science. There is no cure for cancer. If things don't go to plan, you can't get upset. Having two types of breast cancer isn't uncommon, and doctors finding out about the second type of cancer later on isn't uncommon. It's easy to get frustrated because we want to have control, but we don't.

That is one of the things about cancer; it's so out of our control that we just start grasping for straws. It's a waiting game. We live in a state of limbo when in treatment. It's hard to live life when life has to be planned around treatment. I had to get used to waiting for appointments, waiting for doctors to call me back with results, waiting to see what treatment options are available, waiting to heal, waiting for life to start again.

I was already taking Tamoxifen for my estrogen receptor positive cancer, and now I would be taking Herceptin for my hormone receptor positive cancer. Herceptin is a miracle drug for the latter type of breast cancer. If I had gotten breast cancer in the '80s, it would not have been a good time. But now, this drug acts like a cure. Herceptin goes down to the cellular level of the body, finds the hormone receptive cancer cells, goes to that cell and disables the protein on the outside of the cell on the receptors. Basically, it kills them so I wouldn't be affected by the hormones anymore. It requires a treatment of seventeen rounds every twenty-one days. I went to the same chemotherapy room that everyone else goes to, but instead of IVs, I got a drip bag. It was not a walk in the park.

What I didn't anticipate was how hard the treatment would be on me. Because it wasn't chemo, I thought I would just get an IV every three weeks and move on with my life. But the drug made me so tired, I couldn't carry on with my work and my life.

The downside to Herceptin is that it's terrible for your heart. Because of that, I was asked to become part of a study regarding its effects. Every couple of months, I would get an MRI on my heart, and they would monitor me to make sure I could tolerate the drug. At some point, I had to go off of it for about a month to give my heart a break. They measured the ejection fracture rate of my heart, which is basically how hard my heart is pumping. When I started I was at 60%, which was normal. But then it dropped down to almost 40%. That was too low, so they took me off of it for a while before going back on it again.

I was glad that the study provided an extra set of eyes on me watching my health, as well as the Cross staff, when I was getting treatment. It was devastating to know that I'd have to keep going back to the Cross every three weeks for another year, going to the same chemotherapy rooms, even though I wasn't getting chemotherapy. I still had to take a drug that was hard on my body, but it did save my life. The results of that test group changed the way they administer that drug around the world. If a patient gets Herceptin now, they'll be given heart medication along with it. I'm proud to have contributed to that study and hope others' lives will be saved as a result.

Chapter 8:

Bloody and Bandaged, but Beautiful

By the time I finished with chemo, the mastectomy, and radiation, I figured I was in the homestretch and that it wouldn't be long until I'd have my reconstruction surgery. In reality, I had to wait for a consultation with a plastic surgeon, which took about a year. Then, once I got in to see the surgeon, I had to wait another year because my body had to heal substantially after radiation before undergoing the surgery.

One thing I recommend to breast cancer patients who are thinking about reconstruction, at least in Canada where there's a waiting list, is to get on the waiting list even before they're sure they want the surgery. They can always change their mind if they decide they don't want it, two years down the road, when it's actually time to have the surgery.

The night before I was to have the reconstructive surgery, I lay in bed ruminating about it. This was a much more major surgery than my mastectomy because they would have to reconstruct my chest. This was when I was to have my right breast removed, in addition to latissimus dorsi flap reconstruction back surgery. During the reconstruction surgery, an incision is made in the back near the shoulder blade. Then, a patch of skin, fat, blood vessels, and muscle is slid through a tunnel under the skin to the chest and formed into a breast shape. The blood vessels are left attached to their original blood supply in the back; if any blood vessels have to be cut, they are matched to blood vessels in the chest and reattached. Some people get implants as well, which would then be inserted. I wasn't going to get an implant right away. First, I was to get a skin expander, which is kind of like a balloon that they fill with saline about every week until it gets filled.

I had heard horror stories about this surgery. It's an eight-hour surgery that would require a five-day hospital recovery. I would have wounds on my back and front that would take two to three months to heal, and I wouldn't be able to lie down. It was a very hard decision to have the surgery.

Again, I asked myself, *Do I need breasts that bad? Do I care?* And part of me thought, *No*. But then I thought *You know what? I'm young, I don't know what's in front of me. Maybe I won't be married to Mike someday. Maybe I'm going to be single again. I don't know*. I still wanted to look like a sexy lady for myself, so I decided to do it.

I thought the plastic surgeon would be the one to remove my breast, but in the end a general surgeon did it. The general surgeon tried to talk me out of having the second breast removed, but when I told him the conversation I'd had with my original general surgeon, he could see that I'd made up my mind and agreed to move forward.

After waking up after my first reconstruction surgery, the nurse came in and said, "Do you want to see?" I looked down, and even though I only had these two, tiny little mounds that were like the beginning of breasts, I had a moment where I thought, *Oh my god, I feel so pretty!* They were bloody, bandaged, and creepy, but I thought I looked amazing. I realized how much I missed having breasts and the femininity they made me feel. I loved them, and I was so glad I'd made the decision to have the surgery.

It took seven separate surgeries to reconstruct my breasts. Skin expanders were put in, then had to be taken out and traded for implants. The one implant I had was a textured implant, so they took that out and put a smooth one in. Textured implants have been taken off the market since I had my first reconstructive surgery. Studies have found that in a small portion of patients, they can cause another type of cancer. My plastic surgeon decided to take it out and switch it to a smooth silicone implant. I had fat grafting done, which is basically liposuction on my abdomen, then they fill in the gaps to remove the lumps and bumps and make the breasts symmetrical. Using my own fat is a lot better than using an implant so that they look natural and symmetrical. I wanted breasts that look real and fit my body.

Then they built my nipples by folding some skin so I'd have an actual nub, but the areola— where the color is—I wouldn't get back so I had tattooing done. I had no feeling there anyway, so I didn't feel the needles from the tattooing process. Looking at my chest now, someone would know something's happened, but not necessarily that I've had both my breasts taken off. It doesn't look like they're not real. It's quite amazing what surgeons can do.

The Aftermath

Although I no longer have sensation in my breasts, the sexual experience they provide my husband is the same. To him, they look like sexy breasts. The fact that they look symmetrical and real is what is important to him. Again, this is where open communication between partners is key. If you're not ready to have an honest conversation with your partner, then know that you have to have that conversation elsewhere.

There are psychologists and breast cancer support groups available. I recommend that if one support group isn't the right fit, try another. To be real, there can be just one person in a group that wrecks the whole experience. Talk to someone who has had the surgery already. I was fortunate that my chemo buddy went through the mastectomy and reconstruction surgery before I did. No one's cancer experience is the same as anyone else's, but it did help to hear from someone who had gone through what I was about to go through. And she made me an incredible care package right before I went in with a mug, water bottle, trashy magazines, and a nice note!

Breast reconstruction surgery isn't for everyone, but for some women, and certainly for me, it was what I needed to get my confidence back, to get back to real life. Sometimes, it's the last step in closure that breast cancer patients need. It was for me, and I'm really glad I did it. It was a step I needed to put myself back together.

Chapter 9:

Professional and Social Support

After two years of treatment, I had a party. I felt like I had to, like it was what I was supposed to do after beating cancer. Some friends came to my house, and we celebrated. But in truth, I didn't feel like celebrating. I felt like I should feel more excited. I didn't consciously realize it at the time, but I was waiting for the other shoe to drop. I was waiting for cancer to come back, for doctors to tell me that maybe they didn't get it all.

I thought I should be living every day like it was my last, so I was trying to get through my bucket list. I decided I was going to take up dancing. I joined a lyrical class for adults. It was way too hard for me. My head was in a spot where I wasn't sick anymore, but my body was not doing what my mind thought it could do. I didn't altogether realize the affect Herceptin was having on my body. I thought I was done with treatment and I could get on with life, but I couldn't fully.

I also went on a trip to Europe with a girlfriend. We went to Paris and saw the Louvre and the Mona Lisa. We traveled to Versailles and did some things I never thought I would do. I never thought I would see the Eiffel Tower. I never thought I would hang out in Paris all by myself or go to lavish French parties at night. I never thought I would end up in an Italian villa with my girlfriend's family. Pre-cancer, I rarely if ever traveled without my family. It was supposed to be life-affirming, but something was off. Nothing was making me happy, not even a trip to Paris!

When I came back, anytime my husband and I got into an argument over any sort of small thing that came up, I would immediately threaten divorce. My head was in a space that I couldn't navigate alone. I thought I could, but I didn't realize that I was drowning in so many emotions because I had just experienced trauma. I needed help.

The "new normal" wasn't what I thought it was going to be. After surviving cancer, I wanted everything to go back to the way it had been before my diagnosis. I thought, *I'm still Kristi Sainchuk*. But I'm a different Kristi Sainchuk. I will never be the Kristi Sainchuk I was before cancer because it changed me. It changed how I look at life and my values system. Things that were really important to me before are not as important to me now. Things I didn't think I cared about, I care about now. *I miss old Kristi. She was super fun*.

I thought that after everything, I could go back to work. And I did, but I'd get so tired. By 2 p.m., I'd need a nap. And when I say nap, I mean go to bed for the rest of the day. I wasn't as fun as I used to be because life had became serious. When I went to dinner parties or gatherings, I couldn't do small talk anymore. When they asked how I was doing, I would lie and say, "I'm great, I don't have cancer anymore!" But what I wanted to say was that I was sad I got cancer, mad that it stole two years of my life, and that I was disappointed in the direction life was taking me. I wanted to know what was *really* going on in people's lives. Dealing with the minutia of life became hard.

And again, my body was different too. It felt like it was trying to catch up with my head. I thought, *Okay, in a year, it'll catch up.* But even now, it's been eight years since the diagnosis, and I still can't feel my toes. I still can't feel my fingers. I have lymphedema. I still take naps. My taste buds are not the same. I am the wussiest eater of all time; I can't handle spice because my mouth has never recovered. Fresh ground pepper is sometimes too spicy. My hair is not the same. It's still thick, but it's not the same texture as before, and recently I've started to lose a lot of it again due to menopause. My eyes are terrible. I only recently started wearing glasses. I was told that I have cataracts at my last eye appointment, and I'm only forty-four.

I look at my friends who are my age and see how young, spry, and feminine they look. I don't feel that way sometimes. I feel the changes in my body and the way I look. A lot of people don't know how I feel, because I don't tell everyone. It doesn't define me as a person.

The thing that makes cancer not define me is that when I meet somebody, it's not the first thing that comes out of my mouth. It will be weeks or months later when I'll say something about having breast cancer, and they'll look shocked and say, "I never would have known."

I say, "Good, because I don't want Breast Cancer to define me."

People who knew I had cancer still looked at me like I was dying. They treated me differently. It took me a while to realize it, but people were being overly kind to me because they thought I was still sick. I'd say, "I'm fine. I'm done with cancer." But it wouldn't change anything. Once you've had cancer, people still think you're at death's door. I don't think of my life like that, but other people do.

Life did not go back to how it was before, no matter how much I wanted it to.

Breakdown at Costco

After my two years of treatment, the state of my mental health started to become very apparent to my husband Mike in particular. I would sit down with him and say, "I can't handle this for one more second. I didn't fight so long to feel like this. Everything should be perfect now and happy because I finished cancer."

I got into a huge fight with my parents, and then with my brother. I'm not a confrontational person; this was not me. I was angry, belligerent, and awful. If you asked my family what I was like, they would say I was not a happy camper. If you asked anyone else that knew me, they had no idea. I was covering it up.

But I didn't see any of this myself until one day standing in the check-out line at Costco. We have all experienced that line with eight people behind you, everyone with pallets of toilet paper, seven loaves of bread, and a year's supply of dog food. I looked over at the next person and their cart. I saw that level of consumerism and something snapped.

I turned to my husband and asked, "Is this what I fought so fucking hard for? To come back to suburbia every two weeks and buy fucking Goldfish? Is this what life is about now?" I was crying.

He turned to me and said, "I think you better go to the car." I left the store in a messy heap. He paid for the groceries, came back out to the car, took me to 7-11, and promptly bought me a Snickers bar, hoping it would help.

I was calming down but still crying. He said to me, "I really think you better go talk to somebody. You're not doing well." That's when I knew I needed to get help.

I made a call the next day. At the Cross Cancer Institute when I was diagnosed, they told me about all of the services I could access. If I needed financial help, psychological help, or spiritual help, there a program or service for me.

That's where I found the Department of Psychological and Social Services, or Spiritual Services. I had been given the name of one particular doctor from my prior psychologist, who came highly recommended. Her name was Dr. Jill Turner. I reached out to her and said, "I need an appointment. I don't think I'm doing well."

If you're even thinking about seeing a psychologist, you want to make moves to book an appointment sooner rather than later, as wait times can often be several weeks. Similar to the pain medication, you want to get in before you need it.

The Costco incident was a year after my radiation and roughly three or four months post-treatment. I didn't really consider my last year with Herceptin as treatment, but of course it was. It just wasn't chemo. I thought I was done, but this goes back to my previous point that cancer is more complex than you see on TV or hear about.

She made me realize that what I was feeling was very common. I was having trouble with the minutiae of life. I was having trouble with the fact that I still have real life to deal with, such as going to pick up my kids after school, going to Costco for Goldfish, walking the dog, taking out the garbage, and doing everyday stuff. I survived cancer, and now I am scrubbing a toilet.

She told me I couldn't be doing my bucket list every day. I can't be living every day like it's my last because I still have to keep my family and my life going. It was nice to have somebody there that said, "You're okay. It's okay to feel like this." I thought I should just be happy to be alive, and that is not necessarily the case when you're done with cancer. It's hard to just be happy to be alive because now I've had this traumatic thing that's happened to me, and I don't know how to deal with it.

I was so blessed to have my psychologist in my life. I told her I went to a dance class, and I started painting again. I told her I like being creative, but none of these things were making me happy. She said, "Well, you need to figure out what makes you happy now. Everything is going to be new to you. You may think you like coffee because you did before. Taste coffee. Is it really what you like now?" So I started doing that with everything in my life.

I knew I needed an outlet to process all my emotions, and my therapist and I worked through many of them. She told me it was okay to be angry and it was okay to be sad. I had been so incredibly depressed about being really, really sick. Through her I understood that all of my emotions had a place and all of my feelings were valid.

One of the hardest things for me was to let people know when I wasn't okay, that I wasn't feeling great every day, and that I had a mask on a lot of the time when I was sick. I learned that it's okay to be honest. Going to see a therapist saved me in a lot of ways.

NEW PERSPECTIVE: DR. JILL TURNER

Dr. Jill Turner is a clinical psychologist and supportive care lead at CancerControl Alberta for the northern half of the province. Previously, her primary role as a psychologist was seeing inpatients and outpatients.

I see Kristi's Costco incident as not an unusual experience for a lot of patients in our department. We see a lot of people during diagnosis, treatment, and frequently after treatment is completed. Family and friends have a fairly significant expectation for patients that when their treatment has finished, the experience of cancer has finished. For a lot of people, that's when the emotional experience can come to the surface.

When people are in treatment, they have a medical team around them. They're being checked in on, and they have a lot of support people bringing them food and offering to help. There's always somebody on the other end of the phone to answer questions, to lend support and offer reassurance. And then after treatment, it can feel like a very significant transition with a lot of questions about what is next, who is part of their support system, and what does this all mean? All of a sudden there's space and time to think about everything that happened and what it means going forward.

Treatment takes up a lot of time and a lot of mental energy, and patients can spend a lot of their days focused on side effects, medication management, and doctor's appointments. And then when treatment is finished, it can feel like there is a void. That's when heavy emotions can come up. A lot of patients can be caught off guard by the anxiety or fear that bubbles up to the surface when transitioning away from treatment. Sometimes that happens in ways and places we don't expect, like in line at Costco.

Being diagnosed with cancer is abnormal. But for the most part, all of the feelings that happen within that experience are normal. Before a cancer diagnosis, we're allowed to have a lot of emotions. We're allowed to feel anger; we're allowed to feel joy. We're allowed to feel sadness, disappointment, fear, and happiness. But sometimes when people are diagnosed with cancer, there's a lot of pressure to be positive all the time, to be superhuman in terms of coping. If you're in this position, it's important to be kind to yourself. Recognize that you are human and will have a range of emotions and reactions to being diagnosed with cancer and to going through treatments. And that's okay.

At CancerControl Alberta, our services are open to patients, loved ones, family members, and caregivers. We recognize that there are ripple effects to cancer. The cancer experience can impact everyone in a family in different ways, and supporting the family also helps support the patient. Helping family members and loved ones manage their own expectations, normalize their own feelings, or talk about things that are difficult to talk about helps support the whole family.

For people like Kristi—who got cancer when she was in her thirties and whose life was really full with young children, her own business, and an active social life—cancer is really disruptive. Cancer is always disruptive, but in different ways across one's thirties, forties, fifties, and sixties.

People in their thirties are more focused on building relationships, careers, and families. They're really in a place of creativity, and cancer interrupts all that. That's when people are used to being able to do whatever they feel like doing, and they have enough energy to do it. Cancer interrupts that, making patients feel unwell or profoundly fatigued. They have to make choices about where to spend their energy. They need to create new boundaries. This is when a lot of people, especially women, have to learn how to say "No." or "No, not right now, maybe later."

We always like to see people come to our department early on in their diagnosis, but it is hard at the beginning for patients to know what they are going to need. They don't know how they are going to feel. They think maybe they will be the one that coasts through everything. They might feel a desire to continue doing normal everyday things because it makes a difficult time feel more comfortable and familiar. Oftentimes, people want to hang on to "normal" life as much as possible for comfort, but then realize through the treatment process that they might not be able to keep that going. Perhaps they need to make some big adjustments in life. And that is when they might come to see us.

Maybe they need help reassessing their values and deciding where they want to spend their time and energy, or maybe they've always been connected to their values but just need to live them a little bit differently to make time for what's important in a different kind of way. Those are two very difficult things for many people. We can be socialized as women to be people-pleasers, to say yes, to be nice, to smile, and not be angry or say no. Saying no can feel like we're doing something wrong or being selfish. My job is to try to unteach that and help people appreciate the importance of looking after themselves, of knowing their limits, and of respecting those limits so they can maintain some energy and enthusiasm to do things that are important to them.

For some people, connecting with others who have had a similar experience at a similar age can be really important. They may have a different kind of cancer and different treatment, but there is a shared experience that can be very normalizing and validating.

As Kristi says, there is no right way to cope. There is no right way to live with cancer. Everybody needs to find the way that works for them. A certain activity or talking with others might help some people; whereas, others just need to spend time alone, go for walks, be in nature, or read books. Whatever works for you is the right way to cope with cancer.

I would also add that I told Kristi and others like her not to be afraid to try new things. Having cancer is a new experience, and sometimes we need to find new ways of coping. Maybe our old ways aren't working because the new situation is so different and unpredictable. Reach out and take a risk. Who knew that weaving would be such a profound experience for Kristi. (More on that in a later chapter.) Be open to trying something new, and if it doesn't work, don't sweat it. Don't think that you're doing something wrong.

Patients are often inundated by well-meaning people saying read this, do this, my uncle who had cancer did this, or my sister did that. In addition to trying new things, we need to give ourselves permission to let go of things as well. You only need to do what you feel called to do and what makes you feel good.

Get Help before You Think You Need It

To someone reading this who is going through cancer, I tell you there are support services available to you. Reach out to them. In my case, getting a psychologist and then getting the right medication made the difference for me. I met with my psychologist for two years following my breakdown at Costco.

If I had met with my therapist at the beginning, she might have spurred me on to make an appointment once a month just to check-in, which would have been helpful. Things happen during treatment that people aren't expecting or necessarily prepared to deal with, such as issues around body image, relationships, and sexual health. Sexual health is a big one. One hundred percent of people dealing with cancer say that it is something they struggle with because a lot of treatments are hormone treatments, especially with prostate cancer or breast cancer.

It's also a good idea to find a breast cancer support group before you think you need one. Maybe you are not going to go right away, but you will at least have the capacity to attend if you need it. All of a sudden, little things come up and you will think, *I can talk to my breast cancer support group about this.*

For me, I got stuck in the mindset, *You have cancer; here is your treatment plan*, and I went right in fighting for my life. Once that first six to ten months was done, I thought, *What just happened to me? That was so surreal.* I would see pictures of cancer patients at a hockey game getting special treatment or somebody with a critical or terminal illness doing a Make-A-Wish thing, and I would think, *That's just a wonderful story.* And then I'd realize, *Oh, my God, that's what I just went through.* I didn't think it was happening to me. I was definitely in a fighting mode, and then afterward I had a hard time dealing with what happened.

After survival mode, there is a mental health piece to cope with, the after-I-have-survived mode. That took me to the place of, *I thought I should be happy by now.* One thing I know about survival mode is that a lot of times you don't realize you're in survival mode. Even if it doesn't feel like it, reach out and get support in place for when you do need it.

Breast Cancer Support Group

At first, I didn't want to be part of a breast cancer support group. I thought I could deal with everything on my own. *I don't need this. I have good friends. They will help me out.* But after I had my Costco breakdown, I knew I needed to join a breast cancer support group.

A lot of the women in it were going through breast cancer at the time, and I was a year past treatment but still dealing with its repercussions. The group made me feel like I wasn't alone. It made me realize all of the things I had in common with other women who were going through a similar experience. It also made me realize that everybody's story is different. The group helped me learn what I could do to make myself feel better, and it gave me a sounding board.

There was even a dietician that came to speak with us about what we should be eating.

That's when I realized that it doesn't matter who you are, cancer can get you. There was a lady in the group who had done eight Ironman triathlons, and she had breast cancer. To my surprise, there were four people around my age in my breast cancer support group. I met a couple of really good friends. My chemo buddy even ended up being in that group! But I found many other sources of support as well.

Spousal Support

In terms of having a really good support group, my husband was the first line of support. He was a champion about taking care of the kids, working his job, and paying the bills. But I just wanted him to lay in bed and be sick with me all day. That was what I needed. I didn't realize it at the time, so it wasn't something I ever would have been able to verbalize. In hindsight, I realize what an unreasonable and impossible request that would have been for him to grant me, but I was very angry about it for a long time and believed he didn't do enough. But of course, everything he did enabled me to focus on getting better.

In reality, there are probably some things that shouldn't be talked to a spouse about anyway. My husband was taking everything else on to try and keep the household afloat, so he might not have been in a situation to help me emotionally. The whole experience was really hard for him. He was thinking about me dying all the time, and I was thinking about surviving all the time. When he was not around me, he was probably not doing great. I tried my hardest to ask him how he was doing and be there for him, but I simply didn't have the emotional bandwidth to support him in that way. I had to take care of myself and make sure I was healthy. And even when I would try to talk to my husband about his feelings, he really couldn't talk to me about them. Before eventually going to therapy, he did have an emotional outlet in some of his friends. He would share with them how he was feeling or what he was scared about. When he was afraid of me dying, he could talk to them. We didn't and couldn't talk about this with each other because, honestly, I didn't think I was going to die. I was in survival mode, ready to plow through cancer. Perhaps in the back of my mind, I also thought that if we talked about it, it might happen.

The role of the caregiver is something that needs to be worked on in a relationship. I expected it to be my husband, but it really couldn't have been because he was busy outside the home providing for us financially. We were privileged enough to have a nanny, but she was there to take care of the kids, not me. I should have had people in place who could come in and help, especially on those days when I was feeling off, like on days six to ten of chemo. I had food, but once in a while I just needed soup and felt too sick to make it. I felt guilty for asking people to come over and help me because I was sitting in my room eating soda crackers, being sick. But I was also ruminating about being alone and hungry.

As we have gone through our cancer story, my husband went to therapy as well. He learned that it didn't matter what he did for me, I would still have wanted more. I was selfish as a cancer patient. I wanted it all to be about me, but he still had to go to work and support our family. Life went on for everyone but me. Everyone's life wasn't going to stop just because I had cancer, even though sometimes that's exactly what I wanted.

NEW PERSPECTIVE: KRISTI'S HUSBAND, MIKE SAINCHUK

When Kristi got diagnosed, it seemed like I took it harder than she did. She went through it with the mindset, *I'm going to get through this.* I experienced more doubt than her; therefore, it shook me a little more than it shook her.

One of the main things I wish I would have known when she started treatment was that no matter what I did, there was always something more she would wish I would be doing. The harsh reality of the situation is that getting cancer can make a person seem extremely selfish, although I can't really call it selfish because that person is dealing with their mortality. That's something I couldn't understand fully because I wasn't going through what she was. All I can speak for is my own experience.

From my perspective, it felt like she expected me to be there for her all the time. She wanted me to sit with her day in and day out, comfort her, and give her compassion. But that was impossible. No one could do that. I had kids, a mortgage, bills to pay, and a job to worry about on top of dealing with a wife who's trying to beat cancer. I felt pulled in a hundred different directions with no right way of doing any of it.

Another thing I wish I would have known was that I could have gotten support for myself earlier than I did. It felt like I was getting shit on day in and day out, but I couldn't get mad or defensive about it because cancer wasn't something in our control. However, I could have found someone to talk to about it, rather than complaining about my situation as much as I did. I also could have leaned on other people to do more in terms of driving the kids around, making dinners, or helping out at home or work. Besides that, I don't know what else I could have done differently during the treatment period.

A lot of people think a cancer diagnosis brings couples together, but that wasn't our reality. It could have torn us apart. I'm not going to lie; it crossed my mind what life would be like if I were in Mexico by myself. But I'm not that guy who's going to give up on things when they get tough. Leaving would have been the easy way out. We got married for a reason. Every couple goes through issues, and we just happened to go through way too many in a short period of time.

What I worried about more than anything with Kristi getting cancer was what would happen to the kids if she died. Would they even remember who she was? They were so young. I worried more about them than I did me; the kids would have been pretty devastated not having a mom. I felt we could figure out the struggles we had as a couple. They seemed easier and minor compared to how the kids would deal with everything.

Therapy certainly helped get us through everything, but that doesn't mean every therapist should be trusted or is right for you. When Kristi started taking life very seriously and wasn't able to go out and have fun anymore, it really affected me. That meant I wasn't able to go out much anymore and have that outlet because she wanted me to be with her. One of our therapists said that I should only go out with my buddies one time a month and that should be enough. I wanted to get up and leave right there. Who was she to decide how much of an emotional outlet I needed? Women call that self-care. I needed self-care too.

I certainly compromised the number of times I went out, but I didn't always find an appropriate alternative outlet. I probably drank way too much at the time because it was my only way of coping. For other people that stress might have shown up as infidelity, drug use, or weight gain—any number of other ways.

The turning point didn't happen until Kristi was done with treatment. After her breakdown at Costco, she realized she needed professional help. Then through therapy, she learned how to better communicate her needs to me. Things finally improved when she was able to tell me she wished I would help her more and explained what that help looked like to her.

One good thing that came out of her cancer diagnosis for me was that I went from working seventy hours a week to forty hours a week. I realized that, as a business owner, it didn't matter how much I worked, I still made the same amount of money. But even though

I wasn't working as much, I had a lot to handle at home.

What I would share with people who have recently found out their spouse has cancer is that it is going to be extremely difficult. It's not about you. It is about trying to help someone get through it, and you're going to get shit on a lot. You're going to get talked down to a lot, and none of it is purposeful, hateful, or spiteful. The less you take things personally and try to help that person through this challenging time, the better. I didn't realize that right away, but I wish I had.

Art Therapy

All of the levels of support I received throughout my treatment process were critical to my success beating cancer, but what saved my life was going to art therapy. My therapist kept saying to me, "You should just go do a class. Do this. Do that."

I was like, "I don't think so. None of those things are really my thing." I'd heard of art therapy using drumming circles, harp circles, leatherworking, and writing journals, but those were not things that were up my alley.

Then she said, "I know you don't like commitment. That's one of the things we've decided, but we have a pilot project coming up through the arts in medicine program. It's four weeks long, and it's Japanese weaving."

I thought, *Japanese weaving. Yeah, I don't know this about that.* But my therapist kept insisting, and I decided to give it a try. It was only four weeks, and I decided I could handle that. It's safe to say that this decision changed my life.

Chapter 10:

Weave It Out

I went into my art therapy session for Japanese weaving without knowing who was going to be there. I didn't even know the therapist who was leading the class. Through my breast cancer support group, I met many women and became friends with a few of them. But through art therapy, I ended up meeting some very important people in my life, and I had to be cognizant of the fact that they might not always be there.

The very first day we sat down at art therapy, there were six or seven of us in the room. My chemo buddy ended up being there, but I didn't know anyone else. We were sitting in a circle when the last person rushed in. She was bawling as she sat down and joined us. "I'm really sorry," she said. "I need to be here. My name is Julie, and I'm sorry but I'm a mess. My best friend just died from melanoma, which is what I have."

None of us had time for pleasantries. No time for introductions or small talk. We had to come together immediately to support this woman. I don't know that we did a lot of weaving that first day, but something special happened. We all bonded. I met Marie Butler, the art therapist, and I met Tanya Corbin, the weaver that taught us SAORI weaving. All of these magnificent women were suddenly woven into my life.

The story of Misao Jo, who invented SAORI weaving in 1969, is that she was an obi maker. An obi is the large belt that goes on a Japanese kimono. It is the perfectly woven piece of silk that finishes off these beautiful garments. She was weaving on her loom when one of the strings on her warp, the component that turns thread into yarn or fabric, broke. She decided to leave it like that and continue weaving because it was making a fun, wiggly pattern on her obi, and she really liked how it looked. She finished this piece of cloth and thought it was so beautiful. She took it to a kimono merchant who sold obis, and he told her, "You can't sell this. It's flawed." But she took it to a different merchant who thought it was the most beautiful piece of cloth they had ever seen.

She named her weaving style 'SAORI.' In Zen vocabulary, SAORI is the combination of the words "SAI," meaning everything has its own individual dignity, and "ORI," meaning weaving.[1] With this style of weaving, anyone can express oneself freely regardless of age, gender, disability, or intellectual aptitude.

The idea of SAORI weaving comes from the fact that there are no mistakes and that flaws can be beautiful;

---

[1] https://www.saorinomori.com/eng/en_saori.html

they're what make *life* beautiful. Misao Jo has four different principles that she uses to weave, which function as the base of SAORI:

SAORI's Four Principles
1. Consider the differences between people and machines.
2. Be bold and adventurous.
3. Look out through eyes that shine.
4. Inspire one another and everyone in the group.

One of the ideas behind SAORI is that every flower out in nature isn't exactly the same, but they all look beautiful. I connected with that concept when I was healing because, even though cancer is a horrible thing that might seem like a flaw in my life, it's turning into something beautiful. It's what's making my life beautiful.

SAORI weaving is centered on imperfection. I didn't have to worry about making something perfect. There is no wrong way to do it. There are no mistakes, and sometimes the things we think are flaws are actually what makes it beautiful. The first time I sat down at the SAORI loom and wove was the first time I felt genuinely happy after cancer.

Sitting down at the loom, I felt calm and excited. I didn't know anything about weaving, but I fell in love instantly. I didn't want to get up. I thought it was so fun. I couldn't get enough. When it was announced that the class was over, my heart sank. I wanted it to go on forever. The class was only held for two hours every week for four weeks. I, who had been afraid of commitment, knew right then and there that would not be enough.

I started weaving whenever I could. I took the next group session, along with most others in the class, and we would meet after class. I would go in on days when there wasn't a weaving class and ask if anyone was on the loom. If they said no, I would sneak in and ask to weave for a couple hours. Even though I didn't know what it was doing for me, I see now that I was weaving whatever was in my heart.

Whatever I was feeling that day went into the loom and came out as a piece of fabric, and the result didn't matter. It didn't matter if it was pretty. It wasn't about putting something on my table or hanging something on my wall. It was about getting whatever emotion was in my brain and my heart out of me, so that I could move on. I was weaving out the trauma! I never wanted to stop weaving, ever.

When I first agreed to take the weaving class I thought, *Weaving. Ah, whatever. I don't know if I'm going to like this.* But then I remembered that my therapist had encouraged me to try new things I didn't know anything about. I had no inclination whatsoever to weave, but I ended up loving it. This experience goes back to the concept of the "new normal." I wasn't the same person I was pre-diagnosis, so I couldn't assume that the things I used to like or dislike were going to be the same.

Emotion of Color

Usually when I sit down at the loom, I have something going on with my emotions. I might be in a dark mood or a light and airy mood. When I go yarn shopping I think, *Does this fit into how I'm feeling? Does this fit into how I would be able to weave? Does it inspire me?* I am always on the lookout for yarn. I only buy things that speak to me. I have to look at yarn and feel it, and if I think I could use it for a story in my head and my heart, then I buy it.

My Very Own Loom

I was gifted my very own loom by a close friend of mine who knew how much it helped me. She said she couldn't let me go on not having a loom because I was someone who needed to weave every day. "This is your passion." She said. "This is what you want in life, and I can see that it makes you happy." So, I have a SAORI loom, and I love it. I share it with everyone. When somebody is feeling sad, I tell them, "Come over to my house. You need to weave it out today. Just weave that shit out."

Weaving is also what helped me bond with other women who had breast cancer. We've made many tapestries together with all of our different styles of weaving. For example, Julie would take one ball of yarn and just weave an entire foot of the same color.

Jen would weave in so much thick yarn and pieces of fur that her weaving was thick and chunky. We have been there to support each other, and, although we don't see each other all the time now, we do keep in touch.

I make it a goal every day as part of my self-care routine to weave for fifteen minutes a day. Weaving keeps me in the moment. I find it to be meditative. The repetitive movement combined with the clickety-clack of the loom calms me. I get into the moment, and hours can pass without me even thinking about time. It's a very organic process for me.

When I was in high school, I would do pencil drawings, and everything had to be perfect. I tried to sit down and do pencil drawings after I had cancer, and I couldn't. Everything still had to be perfect, so I would leave everything half-done because nothing is ever perfect. But when using the SAORI method as art therapy, it feels like I'm weaving out all of my emotions. I'm human. I don't always have the words, but I still have the pain and sadness inside. I can look at my weaving and see the story that has happened in my weaving. It's a subjective story, but it's a story. Weaving is a catharsis for me.

I've done other art therapies as well where something that looks like a scribble will end up meaning something when I'm done. I'll think, *Oh, that's representing my pain, my body hurting, or my cancer experience*. With art therapy, it's not about having something to hang up on the wall. It's about getting something out of your system. When I sit down, I just weave. I don't have a specific piece in mind that I'm trying to create.

I donated some of the first weavings I made back to silent auctions to raise money for breast cancer. A lot of my weavings are hanging up in my house. Some of them are table runners. Sometimes I give them to people in cancer treatment to hold onto while they're sick or as a prayer shawl. Weavings are very tactile. People love to feel them. I don't want to create something that is just set aside where nobody looks at it or touches it because for me there is emotion and healing in it. I give them to people that I feel need them. If somebody wants to buy one or commission one, I will oblige, but most of the time I weave for myself. I'd never want to make it into a business because I want it to always be enjoyable for me. I want to do it for the love of it, not because I'm going to make money.

Teaching Weaving

Another way I used weaving as a means to give back was through teaching. I joined Volunteer Services at the Cross about four years post-diagnosis. I would be there weaving, and people would come and talk to me about the loom and ask me how to weave. I would invite them to sit down, and I showed them how to weave. They would do a few lines and be in the moment, almost forgetting themselves.

So, in a very organic way, I became a teacher. To teach SAORI I had to use a SAORI loom and take classes to become accredited. But the best part is, anyone can be a student. I realized even kids could do it. So I volunteered to bring my loom to my kids' classroom when they were in grade one.

The loom I have is a travel loom. It folds up like a TV tray, and I can put it in the back of my car and take it to schools. There are tabletop looms as well, but the ones I use are designed specifically for children and people with disabilities so that the loom doesn't get in the way of the weaving. The idea with SAORI weaving is that the loom should not impede anyone from weaving, so it's made to be very easy. It cannot be called SAORI weaving if you are not using a SAORI loom, but you can use the SAORI principles and call it free-form weaving. The same principles apply. When I teach, I tell people the principles that go along with it and what can be learned from it.

When I teach weaving to kids I always tell them, "There is no wrong way to learn how to do this weaving. There are no mistakes, and whatever comes out is how nature wanted you to make it."

They'll say okay, but then when they start weaving they'll ask, "Am I doing this right?"

I'll say, "You're doing it exactly how it's supposed to be done. There's no way you could make this wrong."

And when they're done and they see what they've made, they say, "This is awesome!"

And I say, "Yeah, you're a weaver now."

Kids that don't normally engage in creative activities or the ones that have a hard time sitting still respond well to sitting at the loom and weaving their story. They love whatever five lines they create in the weaving, and then collectively, the class would make a banner together and think it was amazing.

Sharing weaving and teaching kids that there are no mistakes in life made me feel like there was a reason that I went through cancer, that it was just the way life is supposed to be. Sometimes mistakes can be what make things beautiful. That's the way nature wanted life to be.

I was teaching weaving one time in my son and daughters' grade one class, and I got a phone call from a parent the next day. She told me a story about how her little boy was playing with Legos when he stopped following the instructions and started putting them together in whatever way he wanted. His mom said, "That's not how the instructions go."

Her son replied, "Yeah, Mom. There's no wrong way to do this. I'm just going to do it." She said that was such a good lesson for him.

How wonderful would it be if we applied these principles to our whole lives? There's no wrong way to live our lives, there's no wrong way to parent, and there's no wrong way to do our job. It's all perfect, and however it comes out is the way it was meant to come out.

NEW PERSPECTIVE:
MARIE BUTLER, ART THERAPIST

I started working at the Cross Cancer Institute as an art therapist around 2012. Most of my experience with art was with nature. I spent years fashioning home and garden sanctuary items and furniture from willow and birch trees, recycled barn board, and other items.

As art therapists, we have to know our materials and know their felt sense. The felt sense of a material is what will allow for an emotional connection, and that's what we're going after therapeutically. I knew all the basic materials, but my great love was rooted in the comfort, containment, and sanctuary that can be received from the Earth. To me, that is key for therapy, connection and communion with the Earth.

I really wanted the job as an art therapist at the Cross, but it was pretty strange for me because it was in an incredibly sterile environment, quite opposite from Mother Earth ethics. My job was to work a couple of days a week running the arts and medicine program, which meant doing one-on-one therapy supporting children and young people with a horrendous diagnosis and facing death. Then my other two days a week were spent going into the hospital and doing bedside art therapy. This is where SAORI weaving came in.

I was told that I couldn't bring anything living or natural into the hospital because the bacteria on it could kill someone. All of a sudden, I found myself wondering how I could bring the comfort of Mother Earth, of the feminine, into this place if we can't touch anything living.

I started sitting with that question, asking myself what other feminine textures of the heart and soul could be brought into the environment. I also had to think about things that could be easily taught because the students would be very sick. Their minds weren't necessarily working properly, and their energy was low. I went on a quest and came across felting and wool.

Of course, we have so much history as women with sewing, crochet, and knitting. Felting led me to start thinking about weaving because, as I was researching, I found very simple ways of working with thread. The metaphor of thread is incredibly powerful. In life, everything begins with a thread. DNA starts with a thread. There are many Aboriginal teachings, myths, and legends about the red thread that connects us all and the spider web of life. There is a lot of power in that one thread. When that thread is frayed, cut, broken, or disconnected, that can be an incredibly powerful metaphor for disease.

Everything about cancer—what it does to people, how we treat it, and the incredible isolation and disconnect it brings—can be connected to the thread metaphor. I felt like weaving could be that one thread that could pull people back together, into some sort of community and gathering space. Wool is, after all, a gathering material. The way a thread is wound and spun is through gathering.

Soon after that realization I was at a local children's festival when, lo and behold, I ran into Tanya Corbin. She had a booth there and was doing community weaving. She started talking to me about SAORI, and I invited her to the Cross Cancer Institute to give a workshop. She looked at me and said, "I would like that very much."

Within a very short period of time, she and I started a class at the Cross, and Kristi was part of our first group. That group was powerful. It is rare to have a gathering of women from all walks of life, with varied socioeconomic statuses, philosophies, theologies, and religions, all come together for the purpose of healing. It was an incredibly diverse group, and they just gelled. These women shined together. This group became everything that we try to achieve with art as medicine, in heart and soul.

It wasn't about the weaving as a something to *do*; it was about weaving as a way of *being* together. That is SAORI. SAORI is so beautiful. Traditional weaving is very precise and mathematical. SAORI has nothing to do with that. You start with a thread, and that thread is you. The texture of the thread, the color of the thread, the feeling of the thread goes through the warp, and you begin. We had been given grant money, so Tanya and I were able to buy beautiful wool. I felt so blessed to be able to do that because it was our way of saying to the women, "You are so beautiful. You are the finest."

You should have seen their eyes; "For me? I get to use this?" It brings tears to my eyes. They were so happy to be able to receive beauty without having to do anything for it. You can imagine what a powerful thing that was in the face of cancer, its desecration, and everything it's taken from these women's lives. Cancer takes jobs, relationships, and entire lives. At the loom, this group of women started weaving it out.

We've talked about the metaphors of SAORI. The most significant aspect of SAORI is you cannot make a mistake. If something happens in your weaving, such as a thread breaking, the warp going funny in one direction, or you don't like the way the colors are going together, it's all supposed to be there. It's part of the story. It's not about whether someone chooses to wear it, hang it, or do something with it. That's secondary. It's about the story that is unfolding before you on the loom.

I started to refer to the loom as the backbone of our lives. If you don't have a really strong warp, you're not going to be able to weave your story. I started to relate so strongly to the importance of the backbone and the foundation of our stories. *Who's got us right now? Do we feel held? If we don't, can we feel held by this backbone on the loom before us right now?* We worked a lot with that concept.

"Weave, feet, beat" was the rhythm. You weave. Then you press the pedal feet, and then beat. When the women got into the rhythm, they were rocking back and forth. They got into the zone so quickly. Because they had the comfort of everyone there in the circle, they weren't worrying so much about anything else. They could enter themselves.

In Japan, SAORI is a spiritual movement. It has become a philosophy of life that whoever you are, however you come into this life, you get to weave your story. You are always equal. There's a level playing field with SAORI. The base is we are all in harmony. We are all equal. There are no mistakes.

Chapter 11:

What's Different in My Life Because of Cancer

Giving Back

Being able to help others as a result of all of my experiences is what makes me feel like I got some gifts out of having cancer, not that I'd wish it upon anyone. I have been able to witness how weaving helps a lot of people. A member of the Edmonton Weavers' Guild who passed away from cancer donated a loom. The group of ladies from our first class of Japanese weaving pushed to get it placed in the front room of the Cross. It still sits in that sunroom, where family members and patients alike wait for appointments.

Some women were triggered going back to the Cross. I wasn't one of them, so I would go and weave in that room for cancer patients. I was there to make people forget about cancer for five seconds, five minutes, or however long I could. Sometimes patients would come and sit with me, and I'd teach them how to weave. It made me feel really good when I found out that some of the cancer patients would come down in the middle of the night and use the loom. Anything that was made there was turned into blankets or small prayer shawls for people that were at the Cross. It was a cathartic, ethereal process.

Returning to the Cross and helping people makes me feel like I am giving back to the process. I don't feel there is a reason for everything that happens in life, but there are gifts that came out of the fact that I had cancer. I met some amazing people that I would never have met otherwise. When I volunteer, I make people smile; sometimes it's a loved one waiting for somebody to go through an appointment and sometimes it's somebody who has had treatment and used to weave. They get excited about the loom. Other times, it's somebody's dad waiting for their son or daughter's appointment, and they're just excited to see a new machine they can figure out how to work.

I also give speeches about several cancer-related topics now. I lecture at the University of Alberta to second-year medical students as part of their oncology unit. I talk about cancer, body image, and sexual health. I also talk openly about mental health and cancer because what I've learned is that most people can't talk about cancer, let alone the effect it has on their mental health. There is a stigma around mental health, and the more I can normalize it, the more open people will become to talking about the big feelings that come with cancer.

I also have started going back to school to support my weaving. I would love to become an art therapist, and I have taken some classes in that field at the University of Alberta. Another thing I've learned is that I love school and psychology. I have since taken a break from classes to be home and support my children, but I plan to go back again in the future.

As much as I love giving back, I have to limit the amount of time I volunteer at the Cross or be in the cancer world. I have found that when I am there for too long, it can be too heavy and still feel like too much to bear at times. I still have to take care of myself. One of the things I've realized is that if I don't take care of me, then I can get back into that spot of not feeling so good about life anymore.

Self-Care

After I dealt with most of my cancer psychosis, I stopped seeing Dr. Jill because I felt like her time would be better used for somebody going through cancer treatment. I wasn't dealing with a crisis anymore, so I started seeing a cognitive behavioral therapist who is a general practitioner. We'll call her Dr. Jo. She gave me homework. One day, I was telling her what a typical day looked like for me, and she asked, "Why are you doing so much?" I told her I didn't know.

She said, "It's okay to not do so much. If you can only do one thing during the day, that's okay because that's your capacity." I used to view that as being lazy, but now I know my brain can't deal with that many things during the day.

Dr. Jo suggested I cut half my daily tasks out. She made me realize I didn't know what self-care is. I thought self-care was having a bubble bath once in a while. She started me off with taking three deep breaths every morning, every afternoon, and every evening. Yes, she actually had me schedule breathing into my life.

I said, "Maybe I should take a yoga class."

She replied, "But you're already doing too much!" Self-care shouldn't be about doing more. It should be about taking away, doing less, asking for support, delegating to a family member, or even hiring some help.

Having somebody say to me that it is okay to slow down was a big turning point in my life. Just slowing down that little bit changed the way I live. If I have to work, pick up my kids, drive them to Girl Guides, Brownies, or whatever play date they have scheduled; that can be enough for one day. I know anything more than that can lead to a panic attack or some other stress response, like getting angry and yelling at the kids. I leave a lot of space in my life for me now so I don't have those horrible break-downs anymore.

I do my deep breaths. I drink water. I make sure I walk my dogs. I weave for fifteen minutes a day. I try to eat more vegetables. Nothing on my self-care list is so monumentally big that I can't do it. When I'm checking off all those little items, it checks off the big self-care box. Self-care shouldn't be another thing that adds stress.

After having so many surgeries and so many hor-rible things happen to my body, having something that makes my body feel good became very import-ant. On my fortieth birthday, I went to a spa just out-side of Kelowna. It was uber-indulgent, but I wanted to treat myself. I got several treatments done, such as scrubs, a massage, and reflexology on my feet. I'd had so many painful things happen to my body that I forgot there are things I can do to make myself feel better.

Every two weeks I get a massage, and the first time I went to see my massage therapist, I broke down in tears telling her what had happened to me. She said, "Your body just needs some new messages. It needs to be told that the emergency is over. It's okay to relax now."

KRISTI'S SELF-CARE HABITS

✓ Take three deep breaths three times a day at 9 a.m., 2:30 p.m., and 8 p.m.

✓ Weave for fifteen minutes a day.

✓ Swim once a week.

✓ Enjoy a massage every two weeks.

✓ Say no.

✓ Weigh my options when I volunteer. Does it feel good in my heart, or does it feel like a chore already?

✓ Keep my cell phone away from my bed.

✓ Read instead of watching TV before bed.

✓ Go for a walk with the dog.

✓ Keep my water bottle full.

✓ Do not drink alcohol.

Loosening Up

One of the gifts I've gotten out of cancer is being able to put things into perspective. I am clearer about what matters and what doesn't matter. I worry about little things now that I have control over, like what goes in my kids' lunches, my work schedule, and my timetable. I do not try to please people as much any-more. I realized I was spreading myself too thin before I had cancer. I was trying to do too much, see too many people, befriend too many people, and keep up with being a perfect mom, wife, friend, employee, sis-ter, and daughter. Guess what? There is no perfect. I'm just the way nature intended me to be.

When I first started weaving, Tanya, the weaver, was showing us some of her weaving. There was one piece that was loose, airy, and had so many holes in it, I could see through it. I hated that piece of weaving. I thought it was so ugly. I couldn't stand it.

I realized months and years later that the reason I hated it was because I lived my life so tightly wound with no space for me. That piece of weaving made me uncomfortable. Now, I leave space for me in my life. I don't schedule things back to back, running from hockey to dance, to school, and to work without any space in between to breathe. I can't live my life like that anymore.

I've gotten clear with my boundaries. I'm clear about when my work appointments are.

I don't work Mondays. I don't make an appointment after 2 p.m. so I can go pick up my kids. I only like to work three days a week. I try to schedule myself for just two major things a day. I know not to spread myself too thin. I know now I don't have to try to be supermom every day of the week. We order out more than we used to. Sometimes we have breakfast for dinner, and that's okay.

If I have a day where somehow my new schedule and routine wasn't possible and there are too many things going on, I can turn into an angry, sad lady again. It happens very quickly. I'm very cognizant of how and where time is spent. I've gotten better at saying no. I choose who to spend my time with versus trying to spend it with everyone, and I choose what I care about. Weaving remains part of my mental health and self-care routine.

If I keep my self-care routine going in my life, then I feel better. When I'm not doing these things, I can feel myself crashing. I feel the anxiety start to come up, and even driving starts to feel like a humongous chore. The first inclination that I'm not doing well mentally is when the idea of driving to the grocery store, which is only five blocks away, seems like I'm going on a long-distance road trip. I will start getting anxious, phone my husband, and ask him to do it because I can't.

Then, I'll go back over my self-care checklist and ask myself:

- What am I not doing?

- Am I saying yes to too many things?

- Am I not drinking enough water?

- Am I still taking my cell phone to bed with me at night?

- Etc.

There are all these little things on my list that don't seem like very much, but compounded, they make a big difference in my life.

I've learned that sometimes self-care is the thing you don't want to do. For me, I have no problem going for massages or getting bubble baths. What I struggle with is exercising, and yet exercising makes the biggest impact on my mental health, my focus, and my sleep. It's the one thing I should be doing. If you are reading this, take a minute to ask what is going to make the biggest impact on your self-care, regardless of how you feel about it.

In my breast cancer support group, one of the therapists said that what's important is just that you move your body; however that looks for you, just do it. I told Dr. Jo that I wanted to get healthy and be active, but I wasn't who I used to be. I would try to keep up with my forty-year-old friends who were perfectly healthy young ladies, and I've got a bum arm. It was really hard.

Then she said, "Why don't you just walk your dogs every day? Go for two long walks a day, and let that be your starting point. If you get farther than that, great. If you don't, don't be so hard on yourself."

Yeah, that's it right there. High-intensity interval training, running, or Zumba would be too high impact for me. I have terrible knees, but yoga is great. I realized I had a judgment about yoga not being "real exercise," but that was getting in the way of being active. Exercise could just be healthy movement, like my therapist said. I changed my perspective to the idea that exercise doesn't have to be this hard, painful thing. No pain, no gain? Well, no. No pain.

I also learned that self-care is knowing what I'm responsible for. When my mom got sick with cancer seven years after I got sick with breast cancer, the first couple of months felt like I had to carry the whole thing. My mom never made me feel like this, but I felt like I had to. I thought that because I had cancer, I had to be the one to be there for her.

I did some work on that with my therapist, and she asked, "How responsible are you for your mom's cancer?" She showed me a responsibility wheel. One of the things I like about cognitive behavioral therapy is that they gave me homework. I am a visual learner, and the wheel allowed me to see the concept. It turns out, I'm not responsible for my mom's cancer. I'm also not responsible for her treatment. I can guide her in the ways that are good for me, but I also still have to take care of me. I have two other brothers that can support her as well. It wasn't just all about me.

Relationship Communication

The ways my husband and I communicate have changed since going through cancer. If you've read the book *The Five Love Languages*, you'll understand what I mean when I say every individual needs and shows love in different ways. This applies to the way we need support as well. I learned that my biggest love language is quality time. When I needed support through cancer, what mattered the most to me was having someone beside me to talk things out.

Mike felt like the biggest way he could show love was through acts of service. He kept the family running while I was sick, kept the kids taken care of, and worked so we could pay the bills. Those differences were the things we had to work through after I had cancer because I didn't realize what I needed until later. But now we know those things. So now, if I need Mike to be with me because something is going to be hard and I don't feel like carrying it all myself, I ask him to be with me. When I had my surgeries, I had learned by then to tell him, "I know my parents are in town and they're taking care of our children, so I need you to be at the hospital with me." I'm very specific about my needs. I've learned the tools that I need in order to ask directly for what I want.

Chapter 12:

Who I am Now

Now, eight years after walking through my kitchen and finding a lump in my breast, I know who I am better than ever before. A lot about me has changed, but some things haven't. I still have my dream job as the head fashion stylist, but the way I view my job is different. I used to be in the field because of my interest in high fashion and trends. Now, I realize people don't need to wear the latest fashion, they just need to wear clothes. My job is to help people feel good in those clothes, and that in itself is an important job. I teach people from all walks of life how to dress.

I learned so much about cancer and the cancer world by being in it, and now I feel like it's my job to share with people that they can look good and feel good about their bodies no matter what, even if they're going through something like cancer and even if they only have one breast.

Struggling with illness made me more down to earth. My job is less about fashion and more about helping people through tough times. Most people coming to me are trying to get back into life, like moms who have recently had babies, women who have had an illness, or women who are retiring. There's been a life change, and they don't know where to go. I can help them navigate that change.

My job is important to me, but no longer as important as it was before getting cancer. My priority now is my kids and their wellbeing. My twins are ten years old now. They don't talk about cancer often, but they understand what it is. My daughter once said, "You know, Mom, it's really weird that all of my elders have had breast cancer—you, Grandma Linda, Auntie Judy, and Grandma Sylvia."

I told her, "Just because they got cancer doesn't mean you will. It's just something that happened."

My son might say sometimes, "Hey Mom, remember when you were bald?" (Ha!) There is a comfort there, where they feel they can ask me anything about cancer. It's not a taboo subject.

My husband and I have, of course, gone through a lot. We still go to a therapist to keep ourselves on track as a couple. It is an emotionally focused therapy that is less about trying to fix each other and more about how we talk to one other. Our communication has improved. Our sex life will always be different than it was because my hormone levels are zero, but we have tools to deal with that now.

I've heard women going through cancer say they want to give up on their relationship, but that's often because they have given up on life. They will tell their spouse, "You should just go. I'm probably going to die."

When I hear things like that, I say, "Oh, my God. No. You don't know that. You need that person with you." I feel that what is so difficult for many women who get cancer is that their relationship roles change. Women are typically natural caregivers, and then cancer puts them in a situation where they need to be taken care of. They might feel uncomfortable with that. They might feel guilty, like they're a disappointment to their husbands. The work there is to be open to receiving support from their spouse and to communicate instead of turning away.

Why Me?

Many people who get cancer try to figure out the reason why. For me, the first thought that logically came to me was that I had in vitro fertilization, or IVF, so I had all these extra hormones in me. Maybe that was linked to why I had cancer at a young age. I was taking estrogen, progesterone, and testosterone. There's been research done about the correlation between hormone replacement therapy and breast cancer. That being said, if somebody had told me I might get cancer from having IVF, I still would have done it.

By no means do I think that is what caused my cancer. I'll never know the real cause. It could have been because I ate butter one time instead of margarine or because I drank out of a plastic cup that was heated in the microwave. Who knows?

But after that initial question came to mind, the conversation in my head switched to *why me*? Why didn't my friend who smokes two packs of cigarettes a day, drinks beer, and spends all his time in the sun get it? Why did I get cancer and not him? Why did it happen to one of the nicest, most generous people I know—me?

I'm a kind person, and I would do anything for anybody. You call to ask me to help you move, I'm going to help you move. You call me to borrow a cup of sugar, I am there. There was a lot of inner turmoil. *What did I do in my life to deserve this?*

I came to the realization that cancer doesn't care. Cancer doesn't care who you are. It doesn't care how much money you have. It doesn't care how many friends you have, how good of a person you are, what you look like, or what you grew up like. It just doesn't care. It strikes whomever it feels.

I've been in breast cancer support groups and have seen people that take pristine care of their bodies. As I mentioned earlier, a woman in one of my support groups had competed in eight Ironman triathlons. She was the cleanest eater in the entire world, and she had breast cancer. Then there was somebody who just lived life by the seat of her pants, didn't exercise much, or eat healthily. She had breast cancer. It doesn't matter who you are. It just comes when, how, and to whom it comes.

One of the things that helped me was something my sister-in-law said. When I told her I just didn't know why I got cancer and that maybe it was because I had extra hormones in my body. She said, "You know what? You'll never know why you got cancer unless you were standing under an atomic bomb. For sure, you would get cancer then. But you'll never know why, so you need to stop thinking those thoughts because you're never going to get an answer." She pointed out that it was doing nothing positive for my wellbeing to ponder that question.

I used to be somebody who was always stuck in the past, thinking about things that had happened to me and wallowing in self-pity. Now I don't do that. I have a different outlook on life because I stay more in the moment. If I'm having anxiety, I think about my favorite place, the forest, and I think about five things I can see, four things I can smell, three things I can touch, two things I can hear, and one thing I can taste. Paying attention to my senses gets me back in the moment of what I'm doing. Then I realize I'm okay, and I can move on. In this way, even while dealing with the minutiae of life, I'm able to see that life is pretty exquisite.

My kids are priceless. They keep me balanced; they keep me laughing. I joke about the fact now that I have to go to Costco and buy Goldfish. My life wasn't all sunshine and roses before I got cancer, and it's definitely not all sunshine and roses now. My kids have learning disabilities, and I have had to put myself on the back burner to deal with that. But you know what? I've learned that those things can be amazing too.

There Is No Right Way to Have Cancer

If you have cancer, what I want you to know is that however you're experiencing it or dealing with it is fine. There's no right way or wrong way to go through cancer. Your story is your story, and no one can tell you how to deal with your cancer. It's not a competition to see who can handle cancer the best or who fought it the hardest. Everyone who has cancer is fighting for their life in their own way. It is your decision, however you want to deal with it.

Even though cancer wove its way into the tapestry of my life, it has given me gifts that I had no idea I needed. Weaving my life back together again, I can look back and see the beauty of those moments when I learned to live my life for me, as me. Just the way nature intended.

Acknowledgements

To everyone who's made this book possible, there is no way I can say thank you enough. You're all responsible for the ripples of influence that helped shape me to a place where I can speak my truth and tell the story of my time with Cancer.

Thank you to:
- Karen for believing in elephants.
- Marie for showing me that you are never alone in nature.
- Tanya for teaching me how to weave it out.
- Dr. Jill for listening to me and showing me I can reset my life.
- Wendy for giving me a soft place to land.
- Connie for … you know.
- Melanie for watching bad movies with me.
- Bev for holding my babies as if they were your own.
- Claire for being there, even from afar.
- Donna for showing me I have gifts to give to the world.

- Labsies and Cabsies for making me smile and feeding me.
- Jill and Matt for sharing your home with my parents.
- Chantal for giving me the most important hairstyle of my life.
- Jessica for not getting me chia seeds.
- Jen and Paul for keeping me grounded.
- Curtis and Erica for tucking in my babies when I couldn't.
- Brian for inventing the soy sauce key chain.
- Pat J for keeping me dancing.
- Megan for following her dreams… Goulet
- Todd for inspiring me along the way.
- My weaving crew, Jacquie, Ilene and Crystal, you are forever woven into my life.
- The C Retreat women for helping me realize that I have a story that needs to be told.
- Jim Gregson for giving me hope.
- Dana for bringing beauty to a time of darkness.
- Natasha for making me get in the picture and documenting my time with Cancer.
- Cory and Adam for lending me Julie's voice.
- Banner Sparks.
- The incredible team of radiologists, oncologists, and nurses at the Cross Cancer Institute for taking me from diagnosis to where I am today.
- The Volunteers at the Cross Cancer Institute, especially the ones driving the cookie cart.

- Dr. James Wolfli, the most compassionate plastic surgeon out there.
- The team of talented psychologists and counselors that make up the psychosocial and spiritual resources, Spiritual Care Services, at the Cross Cancer Institute.
- Dr. Noella Lee Pong, my GP extraordinaire.
- The village of moms that took care of me and my children when I was recovering from endless surgeries.
- Auntie Judy, Kate, and Elaine.
- My Ivanhoe Cambridge Family.
- My parents, my brothers Geoff and Tim, Felicia, and my nieces, Abbie and Lilly, I love you.
- My amazing in-laws Bruce, Sylvia, and Sharon.
- Kim for taking notes and coming to my appointments with me.
- Zach, Kailyn, and Cameron for making me smile.
- Jennifer Jordan for smiling at me in the waiting room.
- Julie Crawford for letting me make you cheese toast.
- Michael for making me laugh, even in the dark.
- My kids, Sadie and Noah for always being the roots to my tree.

About the Author

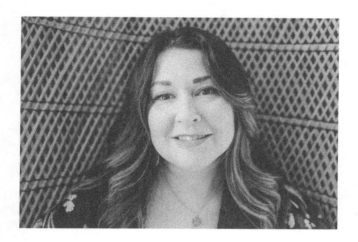

Kristi Sainchuk is a mother of ten-year-old twins, a fashion stylist, and a breast cancer survivor. She was diagnosed in 2012 and has gone through chemotherapy, a bilateral radical mastectomy, radiation, and reconstruction, along with other treatments and bumps along the road.

She has over twenty-five years of experience styling the women of Edmonton, Alberta, Canada. She has a diploma in Fashion Design and Illustration from Marvel College and has worked with several designers in town. After moving into the retail world, she realized that her love of helping women look and feel their best was much more rewarding than designing. As a former owner of a retail store, she developed a loyal clientele of women who relied on her for style advice and honesty. She has styled for various Edmonton TV personas, TV segments, as well as more than fifty fashion shows. Kristi balances her time between being the Head Stylist at Southgate Centre, public speaking, and being the best mom she can be.

CPSIA information can be obtained
at www.ICGtesting.com
Printed in the USA
BVHW081107200620
581838BV00001B/6

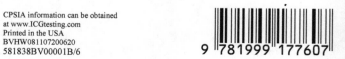

9 781999 177607